LEARNING T
SKIN D

GW01459391

HUMAN HORIZONS SERIES

LEARNING
TO LIVE WITH
SKIN DISORDERS

Christine Orton

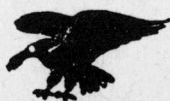

A CONDOR BOOK
SOUVENIR PRESS (E & A) LTD

ISBN 0 285 64945 0 casebound
ISBN 0 285 64946 9 paperback

Printed in Great Britain by
Ebenezer Baylis & Son Ltd.,
The Trinity Press,
Worcester, and London

Illustrations by Ruth Bartlett
Jacket photograph by Richard Denyer

DEDICATED TO MY SON ADAM

Contents

Foreword

Christine Orton has written about the handicap of skin disease. In horse racing a handicap makes it more difficult to win the first prize. In skin disease it is more difficult to win love and money. In sport a handicap is measurable, but unhappily in disablement this is often not so easy. I use the word "unhappily" because, in the World of Science, the consequences of not being measurable are a disadvantage. It often means that the immeasurable is disbelieved and misunderstood. Itching, for instance, is often described as a subjective phenomenon and this sometimes implies that it is "imaginary".

Textbooks of Dermatology are objective and do not elicit much sympathy. One needs books which describe feelings, provided they are well balanced. This book should be read by those whose skin disease is upsetting. It may even help them to be more objective. I hope it will be read by medical social workers and nurses. Perhaps, too, doctors will find it a true reflection of feelings that cannot be written into their own textbooks.

Dr Terence J. Ryan BM, MA, BM, B.Ch., Oxon. FRCP
Consultant Dermatologist,
The Slade Hospital,
Oxford

Introduction

In all there are more than one thousand skin disorders. It is estimated that practically everyone suffers from at least one of these during their lifetime, and that around thirteen percent of consultations in general practice each year are concerned with the skin.

In spite of this, skin disorders are more widely mis-understood than most common health problems. They are the subject of many myths and mysteries, most of which add greatly to the burden of physical, emotional and social problems already suffered by the patient.

A skin disorder can, in fact, be far more a handicap than is generally realised. It can affect how you live, what hobbies you have, what sports you can enjoy. It can influence what you eat and wear; what make-up and toiletries you put on your face and body; how well you do at school and what sort of job you have. It can affect relations with friends, family and the opposite sex and even whether or not you have children at all (since in some conditions there are hereditary factors).

But there are answers to these problems and ways of coming to terms with all skin disorders. We can learn to cope, but this means availing ourselves of all the help available, from correct medical diagnosis to a choice of a huge range of treatments and remedies, from self-help to group therapy, from practical solutions to changes in attitude.

So the purpose of this book is to help people with a skin disorder and their families cope with the effects that this condition will have on their lives, by showing what aid is available. I hope the book will also illustrate to the people who come in contact with them, including those professionally involved such as doctors, teachers and health visitors, how patients feel about their problems and how others can help them most effectively.

The reasons for my conviction that the problems are real and that a book like this is needed are part personal, part professional. Having cared for a son with eczema for many years I have seen and experienced first-hand the sort of difficulties that both the patient and the family have. Even so, until in the course of my work as a freelance journalist, I wrote an article about it all for a national newspaper, I somehow imagined that we were the *only* people to have a problem quite so acute, and that our worries were unique.

But the number of letters I received after the article appeared showed me how wrong I was. They came in their hundreds from parents and patients, all saying how our experience mirrored their own and how they, too, thought they were the only ones to feel like this. Then, through the growth of our own self-help group, the National Eczema Society, and my involvement in preparing its literature, we met doctors and dermatologists and people from other organisations such as The Psoriasis Association and the Skin Disease Research Fund, and realised that many of these problems were shared by patients with other skin disorders.

Yet there were also moments, in gathering the information for this book, when I would wonder whether we were simply blowing everything out of proportion. Talking to a teenager with acne, whose approach to life was admirably straight-forward, and who seemed so little worried by his skin, made me wonder whether after my visit problems would exist where none had been before . . .

Then I arrived home to a letter from a desperate mother whose three-year-old child was covered with psoriasis; and a newspaper cutting about an old lady with eczema so depressed that she had committed suicide. So the need, I felt, was speaking for itself and cases such as the teenager who was coping well would serve to help those who were feeling over-whelmed.

If one is to give an honest picture of the situation it is difficult at times not to sound gloomy and even pessimistic. One constantly has to try to keep a balance between showing how devastating some of the results of a chronic or even mild skin condition can be, and showing how these difficulties can be overcome by the patients themselves and by those they live and meet with.

I hope this balance has been achieved, and that bringing together between the covers of this book as much information as possible on what the problems are and how they can be dealt with will lead to greater understanding for everybody. In the main I have concentrated on what I would call the "Big Three"—acne, psoriasis and eczema—since these are the most common of the longer-term, non-infectious skin disorders. But as the emotional and social effects of most conditions can be similar, where appropriate the rare disabilities and some of the milder ones are included.

I am extremely grateful to the many interested dermatologists, doctors and others professionally involved in the lives of people with skin disorders who have helped provide information, either through interview or through their already published work. My warmest thanks also to The Psoriasis Association and the National Eczema Society for allowing me to draw on their publications, *Beyond the Ointment* and *Exchange*, for information and illustrations. Space permits only a small part of the contents of these magazines to be included in this book, but anyone needing more detailed information about a specific skin condition will find them invaluable. The addresses of the various helping organisations and the names of other useful books to read are listed at the end.

Finally I should like to thank the patients themselves and their families who through articles, interviews and letters have provided the personal experience on which much of this book is based. Particularly, I should like to thank my own family for putting up with the hours of pounding typewriter, and especially Adam, to whom this book is dedicated and without whose suffering I would never have known that the problems I write about existed in the first place.

Christine Orton

1 — Symptoms of Distress

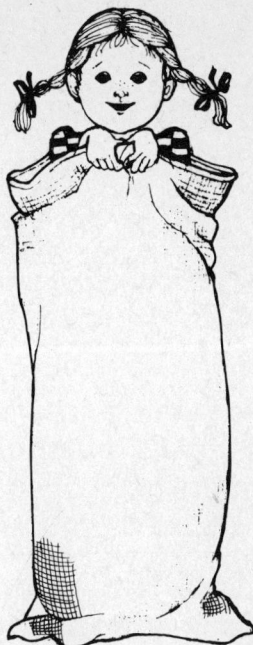

The skin is like a sack that covers you completely

"Please, please, please—somebody find a cure. Not for the eczema, but for the ITCH!''   *Teenage eczema patient*

"Between twenty-four and twenty-five my joints began to get puffy and restricted in movement, starting with my toes, then over a period of some months my neck, ankles, wrists . . . So I sought advice from my GP who passed me on to a consultant, and the disturbing diagnosis: 'It's arthritis, all part of your psoriatic condition.' ''   *Adult psoriasis patient*

"People imagine acne is just a few spots. In fact when the spots are deep and become infected, they can be very painful and sore and cause a great deal of discomfort, physically as well as emotionally.''   *A specialist*

MANY people think of the skin only in terms of appearance, as they smooth in bath oils and moisturising creams, lie in the sun to tan a beautiful golden brown, and shave off excess hair. Men slap on nice smelling after-shave lotions and women highlight their features with make-up.

But in fact the skin has a very practical purpose, and to understand skin disorders it is helpful to have a good knowledge of its anatomy and functions. The most extensive organ of the body, it forms a barrier between ourselves and the outside world. The skin protects, regulates body temperature, helps eliminate waste products, contains sensory organs which act as an early warning system, produces Vitamin D, provides a store of fat and acts as a barometer of the emotions—and all within a thickness of around five millimetres.

At its simplest level the skin is like a sack that covers you completely, keeping together safely all the other body parts. It is made of a relatively tough but elastic material, and is both waterproof and airtight, helping keep harmful substances and moisture out of the body while at the same time controlling the loss of water and other substances from within.

In particular it guards the interior organs against bacteria, its surface an inhospitable desert for invading germs not only because of its dryness, acidity and lack of life-supporting substances, but also because it is constantly shedding itself. In fact if you look at someone's skin everything you see is already dead and peeling away.

In one experiment the skin of a normal hand was found to be contaminated with thirty million bacteria of the streptococci type. But because of the skin's unwelcoming surface, without any further action such as washing having been taken, within one hour the number of germs had dropped to just over one million, and after two hours to below a thousand.

The skin is divided into three main layers. The top layer is called the epidermis and consists of a horny covering of dead cells which are constantly flaking off. The epidermis itself has four layers, and beneath the horny covering are living granular, prickle and basal cells.

In the epidermis, skin cells are formed as a result of cell division in the basal layer. As new cells are produced the older ones are pushed upwards through the prickle and granular layers, changing in shape as they move. By the time they reach the horny layer they are dead cells composed almost entirely of a material called keratin which also forms the hair and nails.

The main function of the epidermis is to maintain and renew the protective horny layer, and it takes about twenty-eight days from the time when a new cell is formed in the basal layer until it is shed from the outside of the skin. The extreme toughness of this uppermost layer is due to keratin, and this in turn is kept supple by the secretion of various glands which have their openings in the epidermis. This suppleness helps protect the more sensitive lower layers of the epidermis against frictional damage.

If the skin is immersed in water for any length of time, the keratinous cells absorb water and become swollen, wrinkling the surface of the skin. On the other hand, when keratin loses its moisture such as in dry, cold conditions, the skin becomes chapped and cracked, allowing the skin barrier to become more easily penetrated.

In the basal layer are special cells which produce a brown pigment called melanin as a protective response to the harmful ultraviolet rays of the sun and this results in the tanned skin which people prize so highly, especially after returning from a holiday. Over thousands of years races living in sunny climates developed extra melanin in their skins as a protection. Races in less sunny parts of the world have had less need for such protection and their skin has less melanin and is lighter coloured in consequence.

Though the sun can have harmful effects on the skin, burning the surface and causing premature ageing with wrinkling and sagging of the underlying tissues, it can also be beneficial for certain skin conditions. Sunlight is also important to a process whereby Vitamin D is manufactured in the skin. Vitamin D is essential to the growth of strong healthy bones, and a deficiency can lead to rickets.

Another pigment which contributes to the surface colour of

the skin is carotene. This is the forerunner of a second vitamin essential to the healthy functioning of the body, Vitamin A, and as its name suggests carotene is a yellow pigment.

The pinkish tone in the skin results from the network of blood vessels which are in the dermis, the layer under the epidermis. The dermis is completely different in structure from the epidermis and apart from the blood vessels it contains various tissue fibres, muscles, nerves, cellular elements and glands. It is really the main part of the skin, with a thickness of around three millimetres, and the skin's blood supply runs through the network of vessels ending in loops of fine capillaries which return to the body's system of veins.

The colour of the skin depends on the amount and state of blood flowing through the capillaries. A fast flow of blood turns the skin pink, whereas a sluggish, deoxygenated blood makes the skin look blue. The temperature of the skin relates to blood flow, too, as the blood vessels contract and dilate to maintain the body in its warm-blooded state. When the blood vessels are contracted the skin looks paler and heat is kept in; when dilated the skin is redder, heat is lost from the surface and the body cools down.

The sweat glands found in the dermis also play an important role in regulating heat by causing heat loss through evaporation of sweat on the skin's surface. Even in a temperate climate such as our own, sweat loss normally amounts to about one and a half litres a day. Ninety percent of this is water, with a major chemical constituent of salt. But on the whole, apart from perhaps when we are nervous or weather is exceptionally hot or we eat something very spicy such as curry, we hardly notice this loss.

Sweating also supplements the work of the kidneys in ridding the body of certain waste products, although it could never take over the function of the kidneys. Sweat contains urea which is a constituent of urine, as well as other substances such as ammonia, all of which add to the distinctive odour that perspiration can have.

Also embedded in the dermis are the hair follicles, little sleeve-like pockets from which hairs appear. By the time we are

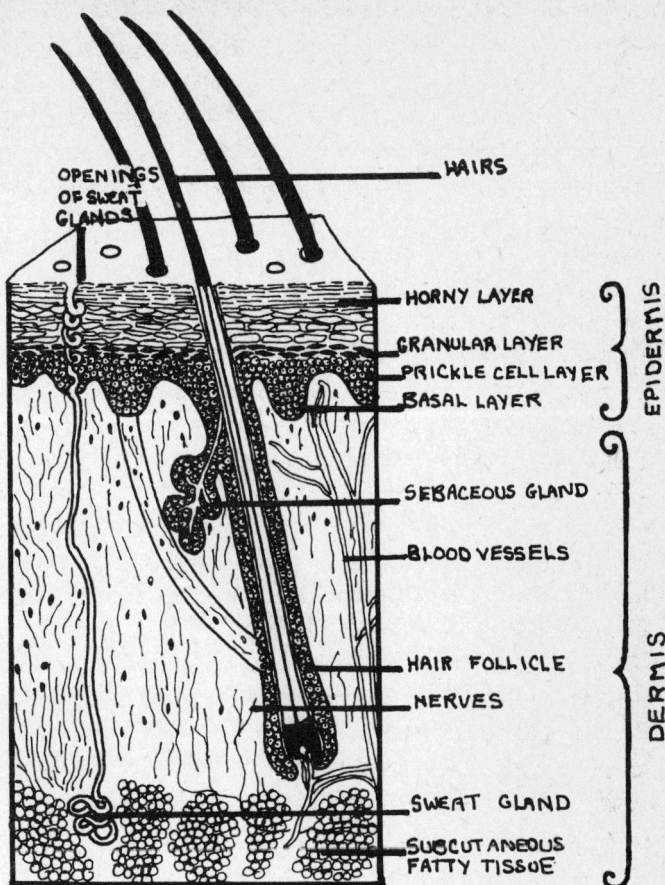

Section of the skin

adults it is estimated that on average there will be about five million hair follicles on the body, of which about one hundred thousand will be on the scalp. All follicles are slanted and a muscle is attached to the middle of each which pulls the hair erect when we are especially frightened or cold, causing "goose pimples". In animals this effect is particularly noticeable, puffing up the fur to make the animal look larger and trapping air in the raised fur which then acts as an insulator.

There are different types of hair, varying in infants, children and adults, and on different parts of the body. For instance, the unborn infant is covered with fine soft hair until the seventh or eighth month when, except for rare instances, it is shed. At birth two types of hair are generally found: a soft, short variety and a longer, coarser one. At puberty all the soft hairs are replaced by coarser ones, which are typically found in the armpits and the genital areas of both sexes and on the face, neck and perhaps chest of men.

Hair growth varies according to the area. The average daily rate on the scalp is around 0.37mm and a hair may grow for two to six years before being shed. The daily growth rate on the male beard is similar. Each hair follicle goes through three phases—first the active, which on the scalp lasts three or four years, then the short phase which lasts two to three weeks and which then leads to the resting period which may last about three months.

The average daily loss of scalp hair is between twenty and eighty hairs, which sounds an enormous amount but which isn't normally noticeable because the surrounding follicles are at different stages of growth. As a dermatologist points out, this figure of daily scalp loss is reassuring to those who may fear that they are going bald when they see hairs on comb, brush or on the basin after washing the hair.

The hair has several functions, apart from adorning the head and looking attractive. It serves as one of the minor mechanisms for regulating the heat of the body and also protects against irritating factors. For instance, the eyebrows are slanted in such a direction that sweat from the forehead is directed away from the eyes; lashes protect the eyes themselves; and the hairs in the nose filter air.

The hair follicle also contains the sebaceous gland, which opens on the surface of the skin. The secretion from this gland, sebum, lubricates the hair. The hair follicle has a luxuriant blood supply and is enmeshed in a network of fine nerves. The nerves supply the muscle, sebaceous gland and the upper part of the follicle, and give great sensitivity to each hair.

The nerve system of the skin is extensive and highly complicated, and on the whole remains another of the mysteries of this most mysterious part of the body. But we do know that nerve endings reach the dermis, and are sensitive to heat, cold, pain, itch and touch. It is in this role as a relay station between external influences and internal organs that the skin plays such an important part, warning us of dangers, telling us whether things are hot or cold, wet or dry, smooth or rough.

The physical reactions of the skin to what we are feeling emotionally or mentally are very obvious. The skin grows pale when we are frightened, hot when we are angry or embarrassed, and secretes more sweat when we are anxious. The scalp will tingle when we are excited, and when stimulated by sexual arousal or affection, the skin—particularly in certain areas—becomes flushed with increased blood flow and highly sensitive to touch.

Such reactions are almost completely involuntary, as are the movements of muscles in the skin, apart from on the neck, and on the face where we have control over expression. Even so, strong emotion can again lead to involuntary movement, such as the lift of a smile, the frown between the eyes or the clouded look of anger.

Various types of cells are also to be found in the dermis, some of which appear in normal healthy conditions and some of which become evident only when disease is present. In health, for example, the white blood cells called the leucocytes act as the body's first line of defence when attacked by bacteria, and lie sparsely round blood vessels. In disease, wherever it occurs in the body, the leucocytes become abundant as they fight the bacteria.

Also in the dermis are the lymphatic vessels which drain away protein substances and tissue fluids, and the connective tissue fibres which bind the layers of skin together. Collagen forms seventy-five percent of the total, and there are also elastic fibres which give the skin its ability to stretch as in pregnancy, and reticulin fibres which ensure stability between dermis and epidermis.

Finally, under both the epidermis and dermis comes what is known as the subcutaneous tissue which consists largely of fat. This acts as a protective cushion for the body and also as a heat insulator, as well as being a reservoir of fat for the body's various needs.

When Things Go Wrong

Like most other organs of the body, the skin goes on quietly functioning away, automatically controlling our temperature, renewing its layers and shedding its dead skin without our noticing much. As long as it works properly, we take it for granted.

But when the various mechanisms go wrong for some reason, then the skin can become a focal point of attention and we don't take it quite so much for granted any more. A cut, or crack, feels sore and opens up a door into the body for bacteria, which is why the smallest injury needs attention and the skin extra protection with antiseptics and plasters.

Boils, spots, blisters or pimples can develop through illness, injury or infection, and the skin can become extra dry or extra greasy. The very preparations we use to make it more beautiful can cause rashes. The skin can become sore and burned by the sun through over-exposure, hairs can grow where we don't want them, hard skin build up on the soles of the feet or the elbows, and wrinkles and lines appear with age.

Sometimes the skin's reaction to emotion can become exaggerated, resulting in constant blushing, or flushing of the whole body surface as in the menopause. Some people develop excessive sweating, which can be particularly embarrassing if it leads to very sweaty palms or an unpleasant smell.

In fact there are hundreds of ways in which the skin can function imperfectly and cause one skin condition or another. Some are so rare that even a dermatologist never sees an example, and others so common that a general practitioner will have regular patients suffering from one or another every week. For this reason it is important that a rash on the skin does have expert diagnosis, since the differences between one and another can be slight yet mean a great deal.

It is possible, for instance, that a rash may be the outward sign of some other illness. Certain ailments such as Hodgkin's Disease, jaundice, diabetes and certain types of cancer may have itching and perhaps a rash as their earliest symptoms. In other conditions, called systemic, the spot, rash or other skin symptom is part of a disorder affecting internal organs too, as in lupus and tuberous sclerosis. (Addresses for special organisations to help with these conditions are at the back of the book.)

Some groups of disorders have certain underlying similarities, such as that they are all inherited. Almost all are variable in the extent to which they affect different people, so that in one a condition may be mild and in another severe. There are also several types of one condition, and certain skin disorders, such as eczema and psoriasis, tend to wax and wane so that the patient will vary from month to month, sometimes suddenly recovering completely for no apparent reason. Damage to the skin in certain skin disorders also appears to affect its temperature control mechanism and sweat loss so that some patients, for instance those with extensive eczema, find that at times they feel hot in cold weather and vice versa. A very sore body can also lead to bouts of shivering, maybe through shock or loss of body heat.

However, all the conditions also have slight but nevertheless distinct variations in symptoms, and hence different effects on our social and emotional lives. And though what actually triggers them off, so that one person comes out in spots and rashes and another does not, remains unclear, the way the normal working of the skin breaks down in any given disorder is more obvious.

Psoriasis is probably one of the most common of all skin conditions, and is thought to affect between two and three percent of the population to some degree. In this disorder the cell renewal process described earlier is speeded up to such an extent that instead of taking around twenty-seven days it may take as few as four. The red or dull salmon pink patches, usually circular in shape, which characterise psoriasis become covered with loose silvery scales which flake off constantly in a fine powder or in larger pieces. These scales consist of both live and dead cells.

This constant shedding of skin can cause the patient a great deal of inconvenience, since clothes and the floor area round bed or chair can become covered with them. Even though creams and special baths can remove them, they renew so quickly that they are difficult to keep under control and create a particular problem on the head where they gather in the form of thick dandruff or a helmet-like crust.

For both men and women patients, this can cause many practical problems in keeping hair presentable, and particularly in visiting hairdressers. Says Ray Jobling in the book *Medical Encounters* for which he has written a chapter about living with psoriasis:

> "Getting a haircut presented a potential problem though this was overcome by remaining loyal to a single hairdresser who proved to be both knowledgeable and sympathetic, to the extent of taking great pains to maintain and even enhance my protective style.
>
> "More troublesome was the apparent affliction by dandruff as a result of the scaliness of the scalp. I learned that dandruff seems to constitute a moral offence in its own right, carrying connotations of personal responsibility and neglect so I took trouble to prevent any suspicion of it."

A woman patient describes how she, too, hates going to the hairdresser because of the questions that get asked and the disdainful attitude that can result. "Even worse is the constant advice on how to get rid of what everyone thinks is a bad attack of dandruff," she comments. "I say that it isn't dandruff and show I have got it all over to prove it, but the only real answer is to find a sympathetic and experienced hairdresser."

Even when psoriasis seriously affects the scalp it usually finishes at the hairline, and it is fairly unusual for it to appear on the face. Psoriasis does not always irritate, but a large proportion of people do suffer from itching. Some find that this is related to treatment, and some irritate more when they are feeling nervous or strained.

In fact, as with most skin conditions, there are few hard and fast rules about the pattern of psoriasis. Whereas one thing may be true for one person it may not be true for another. The psoriasis will vary in its severity, some people having only a few small patches on elbows and knees, others having larger patches involving a greater area of the body. In certain cases the patches have no scaling, though the majority do.

The condition will also fluctuate, and in many cases suddenly disappear altogether, either for a short period or for good. In some people it becomes worse during puberty, pregnancy and menopause, but others may be completely clear at these times. There are also different types of psoriasis, and the extent to which a person is affected may depend on this. In certain cases the patches may crack and become sore, in one type pustules develop and in a proportion of patients there can be a mild form of allied arthritis. It is possible for a patient to switch from one type of psoriasis to another and for symptoms to be linked with treatment.

There is also a variety called guttate or "raindrop" psoriasis which consists of many very small scaly patches on the trunk and limbs and sometimes the scalp. This type of rash often follows an infection in the throat and is a form of psoriasis that can clear quite quickly. But in some the patches linger indefinitely. If the psoriasis is found to return with future attacks of tonsilitis, the removal of the tonsils may be advised.

Psoriasis is neither contagious nor caused by bad hygiene, it affects men and women in equal numbers and can start at any time in life. But this can only be in a person predisposed to the condition and it cannot be "caught" sitting in a train or touching hands as some people still seem to think. Psoriasis is usually inherited although this is not always apparent, and it is thought that where there is an inborn tendency to develop the condition it can be triggered off by a variety of factors, including injury, infection, hormonal changes, certain drugs and stress. Even so, the actual origin of the physical process whereby skin cells renew so fast and red patches appear is still not known.

In *acne* the main divergence from the normal functioning of the skin appears to be a very much increased production of sebum by the sebaceous glands, called seborrhoea, and the severity of the patient's acne is related to the natural greasiness of his or her skin. The gland openings become blocked deep down with a mixture of sebum, hair and dried skin, with consequent infection. The result will be the large, inflamed and sometimes very deep spots of acne, often accompanied by both black heads and enclosed white heads known as "closed" comedones.

Acne appears predominantly on the face, back and chest because these are the areas of the body most freely endowed with sebaceous glands. These glands are also found on the scalp, but this area is protected from developing acne by the presence of the hairs which allow the sebum to drain away without developing any obstruction.

Again, the basic reason behind this malfunctioning of the skin which causes some people to produce too much sebum is still not fully understood. However, it is thought to be connected with the production of hormones, particularly the male hormone which both men and women have naturally in their bodies. It is probably for this reason that acne is so commonplace among adolescents, when the whole body is undergoing dramatic changes.

It is however possible for quite young children, even babies, to develop acne, and also for men and women to have it in their later years, though quite often this succeeds an earlier history of acne during adolescence. There may be a link with hormones in these cases too, due to the general hormone imbalance in newborn babies, and, in women, during pre-menstrual periods and the menopause.

Some people think of acne as so common that they feel it is hardly worth worrying about, and it is true that a very high proportion of adolescents suffer from it to a slight degree. They take a few spots for granted as part of growing up. But, as with other skin conditions, acne can vary in severity and it is when it is really extensive and persists for years in spite of treatment that it takes its toll.

Acne does not irritate, but when it is infected and the spots are deep and prolific it can be very painful and uncomfortable. The temptation is to touch and squeeze them, but this can lead to increased infection and possible long-term scarring. Even when physical discomfort is not so great, there is little need to point out the anguish that the condition can cause the patient because of its effect on appearance at a particularly sensitive age.

Eczema is another condition with a wide variety of manifestations—around fourteen in all—most of them resulting in red, itchy, often weeping rashes on the skin which are intensely irritating. The word eczema is derived from the Greek word meaning "to boil over or break out", and this very aptly describes the skin's appearance. It becomes inflamed and slightly swollen with blister-like pimples on the surface which, particularly if scratched, will weep and become crusted.

There are certain basic differences between the normal skin and that of the person with certain types of eczema. For instance in *infantile* eczema, or *atopic* eczema as it is medically known, the skin may be generally paler than normal and respond to stroking by blanching at the point of contact.

It is believed by many skin specialists that these patients have a low "itch threshold", and what is felt as touch by most people is felt as irritation to them. There is usually a tendency to dryness of the skin, which can lead to sore patches and cracking, and the skin is sensitive to irritant substances and to changes in the weather such as cold and wind in winter, or marked heat and humidity in summer.

It is not yet known how localised is the rash reaction of the skin, or how much due to a problem in another part of the body, such as allergy to food in the intestine. In fact whether atopic eczema is related to allergy at all is still hotly debated, partly because allergy is another complicated mechanism about which there are still many mysteries.

However, it does help for the patient to have an idea of what allergy is and how it may affect the skin. As one specialist explains, basically it is an exaggerated response of the body's immune system which normally protects us from attack by illnesses such as measles, chickenpox or sore throats, but which can react in the allergic person to a whole range of substances from dust to milk to pollen.

Allergen or antigen is the name given to the particular substance which causes allergy in someone; sensitisation is the process by which this allergy comes about; and antibodies are proteins circulating in the blood stream which fight away invading allergen by helping the body cells release a substance called histamine.

In the person with asthma the body's reaction to this release of histamine will be coughing and sneezing, and in the person with hayfever there will be running eyes and sneezing. The reaction of the skin to allergy is thought to be a rather more complicated process, but in certain types of eczema the effect is an itchy and inflamed skin.

Children who have the infantile or atopic type of eczema will often have asthma or hayfever too, but in spite of this it is by no means proved that the eczema they suffer is also the direct reaction to allergy. Even if it is, the person is often sensitive to so many things in the environment that it would be impossible to rule them all out. Occasionally, however, the culprit can be traced, as when babies are taken off cows' milk and improve. More detail about work in this field is mentioned in Chapter 5.

In spite of its name, infantile eczema can continue into adulthood, but adults also suffer very commonly from the *irritant* or *contact* type of eczema (or *dermatitis* as it is also often called). The first is caused by a person coming in contact with an irritant substance which damages the surface of the skin, the second by an allergen actually penetrating the skin and setting off an allergic reaction.

The symptoms are very similar in all three types of eczema, which is where confusion may arise. But whereas atopic eczema is an inborn condition, contact and irritant eczema are reactions to outside agents and can happen to almost anyone. It is also possible for the same substance, for instance wet cement, to be both an irritant and an allergen.

In contact eczema a wide variety of substances can create an allergic reaction in a person's skin. But just to confuse matters, this may happen after years of regular use of the material in question without apparent ill effect, and may not be only at the site of contact. For instance, a middle-aged woman may break out in a rash on her arm which is caused by the nickel bracelet she has worn for years.

Rubber gloves can suddenly cause an allergic rash, and one dermatologist describes how a woman showed reaction to nail varnish on her chin because she was always putting her hand there. Some allergies and irritant rashes are caused by substances people come into contact with through their jobs, such as the resins in plastics and adhesives, and in this case the resulting eczema comes under the heading of *industrial dermatitis*.

Another form of eczema is *seborrhoeic*, which mainly effects the scalp where it has the appearance of rather bad dandruff or cradle cap. Redness and scaling can spread beyond the hairline and over the ears, eybrows and the folds round the nose, and it can also involve the body in the groin, the centre of the chest and the middle of the back. It usually runs a mild, intermittent course, occasionally flaring up but also disappearing completely.

Discoid eczema takes its name from the shape of the rash, which occurs as well-defined, coin-like discs of red, crusted, scaly skin. The legs are usually affected more than the arms and this is a condition mainly of the middle-aged and elderly. Men are sometimes more affected than women. Often mistaken for ringworm or psoriasis, discoid eczema can be distinguished by the yellow sticking scales which are unlike the silvery scales of psoriasis.

Varicose eczema is also usually found in the middle-aged and elderly, especially women. It involves the lower third of the legs (not the feet) and is characteristically associated with varicose veins and varicose ulcers. Overweight and hereditary factors may also play a part.

In eczema the actual condition and the resulting irritation and scratching can alter the appearance of the skin. For instance, after an area of skin has been constantly rubbed or scratched for a length of time, the surface becomes thicker and darker, with a leathery surface. This is known as "lichenification". Also pigmentation in the skin may alter, causing white patches in some and darker patches in others. Finally, eczema can become infected—although like the other skin disorders mentioned so far it is not contagious in itself—and is particularly susceptible to impetigo and cold sores, both of which should be avoided and treated very promptly if picked up.

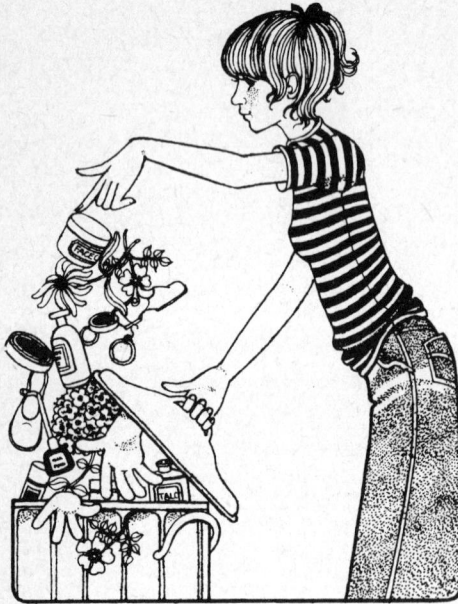

Find out what irritates your skin — and avoid it

Irritating Problems

It is this sensitivity of the skin which causes eczema sufferers so many problems, and though they may not be allergic to certain substances the skin can very often be irritated by them, whether they be make-up, detergents or even certain flowers. The fact that the patient with eczema tends to feel hot leads to further irritation, and cotton clothes and bedding are needed next to the skin.

For many people with skin complaints it is the irritation which causes them most torment. ''The itching really is as bad as being tortured,'' writes one adult eczema sufferer. ''I have eczema between all my toes and under the surface of the foot.

Sometimes at four in the morning wild thoughts of chopping off my toes torment me. In the morning I wonder if perhaps I've been crazy in the night.''

A doctor who had eczema as a child describes how you need to understand this itch before you can understand what it does to someone's feelings. ''The eczema sufferer isn't wilfully attacking an inert skin. He's battling with an incorrigible itch. It isn't the itch of a normal person who feels it on the surface of the skin and stops it by gently massaging the surface. It is in the skin itself, which explains those horrific attempts children seem to be making to gouge it out.

''And it isn't just caused by normal irritants—insects or chemicals, for instance. It may be caused by these, but by millions of other things as well: by contact with clothes or furniture or hair, by specific allergies to foods or animals or plants or dust, by heat or cold or dryness or wetness or worry or excitement or exercise. And it arises out of the blue—spontaneous, unpredictable itching which can build up gradually or arrive like a tropical thunderstorm.''

This doctor explains the complicated range of emotions the person may feel after he or she has given in to a passionate bout of scratching as: ''an overwhelming feeling of futility, unhappiness or shock. This may be complicated by shame at having succumbed once again, by fear of punishment or ridicule or the physical discomfort which is scratching's natural sequel. This peculiar physical and emotional conflict, then, is your everyday experience.''

Nowadays many people come to terms with the problem by following the advice of dermatologists who recommend scratching, without feeling guilty, whenever you need to. The theory behind this is that in the end you scratch less, especially at night when otherwise there is a build-up of the urge and no conscious control.

Views among specialists vary on this point, but there are certainly many doctors who agree that this is the right attitude to take, particularly with children. It can, however, lead to further social problems in that there may be blood stains on clothing and bedding. The skin may become so sore that it is difficult to carry out certain tasks, making even walking difficult and bathing the baby or washing up impossible. It can also be very hard for others to look on and see a person scratch without trying to stop them!

Eczema, and in particular contact and industrial eczema, can also have a profound effect on a person's job if he or she is reacting to something closely allied to it. A career change may be necessary in some cases, although usually it is possible to find a way of avoiding the guilty substance. One girl, for instance, who was sensitive to the ink used in an old fashioned copying machine changed to an office with more up-to-date equipment and her eczema disappeared.

Urticaria is another allergic condition and can be confused with eczema since it shows itself in a red, swollen itchy rash on the skin. Also known as welts, hives, nettlerash or contact wealing, the inflamed area may have a raised whitish centre which gives it the appearance of a mosquito bite. Urticaria is often the immediate reaction of the skin to some contacted, inhaled or digested substance to which the sufferer is allergic, from a wasp sting to a plate of fish for supper. Urticaria is also made worse by overheating, hot baths or showers, emotional upsets and pressure such as that from a tight waistband or bra strap.

On the whole it is not a long-term condition, most adults and children experiencing it only occasionally. But there are some for whom it can be a major difficulty when the rash lasts for months on end and even years. Some, too, have internal swelling (called oedema) of tongue and throat so that breathing can be affected. This has to be carefully watched, especially in babies who may have a violent allergy to eggs or some food they have not tried before.

It is also possible to have urticaria in combination with another skin condition such as eczema, and this can add great complications, the symptoms of one confusing those of the other and the general irritation becoming even worse.

Pruritis is the medical name for itching, but is often used when speaking of irritation or rashes in the genital area—"embarrassing itching", as it is described on occasion!

As will be seen in future chapters, this has been put down in the past to psychological causes but in fact is often due to specific skin conditions, infection, or worms.

There may be candida or some other bacterial complication present, or an allergic reaction to a contraceptive. Other skin conditions such as eczema and psoriasis can be particularly virulent in these areas and pruritis can also come about through dry skin, pregnancy and the use of certain drugs. Itching can also be the symptom of some other illnesses, and it is important that it should be mentioned to doctors rather than ignored as a nasty but trivial part of life.

Icthyosis is another skin condition which can combine with something like eczema, increasing the symptoms. It is generally hereditary and the skin is extremely dry and scaly—hence the nickname "fish scale disease". It is thought that it may be due to some abnormality in the production of keratin in the horny layer of the epidermis, so that, rather as in psoriasis, the shedding of the dead cells from the surface is speeded up. The skin does tend to crack, but though there are some extreme cases where the whole body is badly affected, in most people icthyosis can be kept under control with lubricants and moisturisers.

Rosacea would seem to be a congestion and dilation of the blood vessels in the face, especially on the nose and cheeks, resulting in a permanently flushed appearance, often with some acne-like spots and dryness. In the early stages there may be exaggerated flushing of the skin in response to food, heat and emotional stress, and later this flush appears to become permanent, with red veining on cheeks and nose.

It can be a particularly awkward skin condition to suffer from as it will give the impression of social unease even when none is felt, and a flushed face tends to draw attention and comment from other people which is the last thing the patient wants. Another unfortunate side-effect of rosacea can be a very red and swollen nose, which may lead to suspicions of alcoholic over-indulgence!

Alopecia is the overall name given to sudden loss of hair, either in small patches on the scalp, or so extensively that the patient loses eyebrows and hair from other parts of the body. The complaint is common in childhood and can be very worrying for parents as well as difficult for the child. But unlike the baldness found in men, in most cases of alopecia the hair regrows. The condition may occur after a serious illness or some traumatic shock, or even be caused by certain hairstyles, such as the pony tail, which put strain on the hair.

At the other end of the spectrum comes superfluous hair, or *hirsutism* as it is medically known. This can vary from an unwanted growth on a woman's face to an extensive amount in other parts of the body. The cause appears to be a matter of constitution, hereditary factors, and hormonal growth and development. Some cases are associated with glandular disorders, menopause or even side-effects from drugs. Excess hair can be very distressing, and again it is important not just to put up with it but to research the various methods of removal.

Some skin problems are due to faulty pigmentation in the skin. In *vitiligo*, for instance, pale areas develop on parts of the body, most commonly on the face, neck and hands. Those suffering this condition discover that the pale areas are very sensitive to sunlight and if exposed to it for any length of time become red and painful.

Sensitivity to sunlight, or *photosensitivity*, causes a whole range of skin conditions including a type of eczema, and is different from the blistering and burning reaction which many people have after exposure to the sun. Certain patients, for instance, can hardly expose any part of their body without coming out in an itchy rash or skin eruption, and certain drugs make this effect even worse. This can have crippling results, since the sufferer must either hide from sunshine altogether or wear clothing to cover all parts of the body.

Naevi, or birthmarks as they are commonly known, are another form of faulty pigmentation. In this case there is an area of darker staining of the skin as in the port-wine stain which will often appear down one side of the face, or a bright red swelling which can appear on any part of the body, known as a strawberry mark.

This latter type is found in about ten percent of all babies, and will usually clear up by the time the child is five or six. But extensive birthmarks of the port-wine type present a more long-term problem and are sometimes dealt with by plastic surgery or special cosmetics.

There are other varieties of skin conditions, including those which cause blistering such as *epidermolysis bullosa* or hardening of the skin and internal organs as in *scleroderma*, which can have a drastic effect on people's lives. These are thankfully rare, but common enough for self-help groups to have started to support the sufferers and their families (addresses at the back of the book).

In fact the list of skin conditions could be endless, including the common fungal disorders such as ringworm, the virus infections such as cold sores or warts, the infestations like scabies or infected rashes including impetigo. But since most of these are short-term and curable, they do not usually cause the sort of social and emotional difficulties of longer-term disorders and as has already been explained are not on the whole the skin conditions this book aims to discuss.

They may, however, give the sufferer some insight into just how devastating a condition that doesn't disappear easily can be. "It is like so many things in life" writes one man. "Until it happens to you, it is not of major importance. When it does happen, one wants help from anyone who can offer it. Likewise we should be willing to help anyone among us who needs help."

The good news is that, depressing reading though the long list of skin disorders and their symptoms in this chapter may make, there are sources of help available in coping with them. To know something about the effects that a disorder may have can help a person learn to live as fully as possible in spite of them, and also help others be more sympathetic.

For instance, if the teacher at school knows that itching is a very real part of a child's eczema and not just something he puts on to gain attention or to get out of certain lessons (as has been thought on occasion) energy can go into helping the child cope rather than into telling him to pull himself together. If hairdressers and people in the street know that scales are a natural part of psoriasis, they are not going to be so worried by them. If people know that acne is a result of hormonal imbalance they are less likely to hint that cleanliness might be the answer, and the patient is less likely to start washing obsessively.

Many patients anyway, find that, having accepted certain limitations caused by their condition, they can still live the lives they want to live. One thirteen-year-old I know with asthma and eczema won a three-mile cross country race and represented his school at county championship level. A psoriasis patient describes how he has been a physiotherapist for numerous ice hockey teams: "Forget your spots and they may forget you", he says.

The patient quoted at the opening of this chapter, who developed arthritis, adds: "Fear not, those with poly-arthritis, the wheelchair vision never materialised. Far from it. One of my early ambitions was to fly an aircraft and I did. I actually obtained a Private Pilot's licence at the local flying club in the midst of my arthritic condition."

Others find the answers lie in practical measures, such as taking disposable sheets or bedding away for weekends and holidays, or using cotton gloves for certain jobs when the hands are very painful. One woman with acne took up sport because she felt the open-air life might help the condition—and ended up meeting her future husband.

Armed with the correct information about your condition and a basic understanding of the symptoms, you are in a much stronger position to distinguish between what is fact and what is fancy, and to be less influenced by other people's misconceptions about skin disorders. You can then take the first steps in planning life so as to minimise their effects.

In later chapters we shall discuss general attitudes to skin disorders, and the emotional and psychological approaches to them as well as the sort of measures that can be taken to make life easier for the baby, the growing child, the adolescent and the adult. But having diagnosed the condition the next step is to find the correct treatment that will control symptoms until, perhaps, the disorder clears of its own accord.

Read on and you'll hear more about them.

2 – A Suitable Treatment

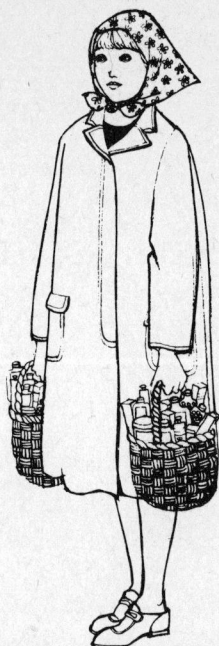

Armed with lotions and creams, tablets and ointments, it is mostly for the patient to treat himself

"I feel very strongly that psoriasis is an ailment that one must come to terms with, and, therefore, that treatment must be personally and socially acceptable. I have so far been given ointments that without exception either smell highly and/or are very greasy and/or stain the skin . . ."

Man with psoriasis

"There were times when I longed for a break from the bedtime routine. If only, through the many years she had eczema, I could have handed over the creaming, bathing and bandaging just occasionally." *A mother*

"I remember as a teenager being told to leave my spots alone and they'd go away. But they didn't, and now I've got the scars to prove it." *Bruce, aged 40*

RECOMMENDS one medical compendium of 1825: 'To "To control the itch mix your own sulphur with fresh butter or lard plus a few drops of oil of lavender to conceal the disagreeable smell. If severe itching and irritation continues, apply four leeches . . ."

Treatments for skin conditions have come a long way since those days. The majority of preparations come ready-packaged and odourless, some to be bought over the counter from the chemist and others through a prescription from the doctor. In certain cases treatments, if used correctly, are now so successful that a disorder which once might have led to months or even a life-time of discomfort and unsightliness can be brought under control almost overnight.

Many people do not even go to the doctor with a rash, preferring either to wait until it goes away or perhaps to try some proprietary brand of cream. In fact self-medication in skin disorders is very common and one survey showed that of twenty-two percent of a sample of people interviewed who had experienced skin complaints in the previous two weeks, about one half had medicated themselves compared with about a sixth who had taken medication prescribed by a doctor.

Another survey showed that apart from analgesics, skin preparations are to be found in a higher proportion of homes than any other type of medicine. Forty-eight percent of households kept simple skin creams such as balms, oils, anti-pruritics and local anaesthetics at the time of interview and the majority of items whether in use or not were non-prescribed.

Says a report by the Office of Health Economics:

"There is a very wide range of medicaments available over the counter for skin complaints although there may be some doubt as to whether some are properly termed medicaments or whether they should be classified as toiletries or even cosmetics.

"For example, it may be difficult to define, except by some arbitrary rule, where a medicated shampoo properly belongs. It may be used as part of the normal toilet and this arguably should not be considered self-medication, but on the other hand many medicated shampoos do contain compounds which are at least partially effective against some scalp conditions such as dandruff. Furthermore, soap whether it is medicated or not has in itself an important part to play in the prevention of such skin conditions as acne.''

But even though self-medication may be popular in treating skin conditions, and very often through trial and error the patient can hit upon some particular cream or remedy which does the trick, it is vital to seek professional diagnosis if any rash or irritation on the skin lasts longer than a few days.

For instance, the dandruff which persists may turn out to be part of the wider symptoms of seborrhoeic eczema which also affects the chest, nose and ears with itchy patches. And as we have seen from the last chapter, in some cases this could be a symptom of psoriasis where scaling often involves the scalp.

Just as important even though there may be only a slight difference between one rash and another, there can be a world of difference between suitable treatments and it will take an expert to pick this up. Surprising though it may seem, scabies has been mistaken for eczema, and the treatment for one could make the other a great deal worse.

Similarly, though steroid preparations may help certain skin conditions, they can cause others such as rosacea to spread even further, and when infection is present in a condition such as eczema the steroids need to have the addition of antibiotics. One boy was thought to have eczema, but when the blistering disorder *dermatitis herpetiformis* was diagnosed a non-gluten diet cleared the rash.

Even within the same skin condition, different types will need a separate treatment or approach. The rashes of atopic eczema and contact eczema may be alike. But whereas the use of creams may suppress both rashes, particularly in the latter case it is possible to seek out the cause and avoid it so that the condition is cured completely.

It is also possible to go on suffering from a particular disorder when a visit to the doctor and an accurate diagnosis could clear the problem up. Use the right treatment for the right rash and the symptoms could disappear altogether, at least as far as the eye can see.

For all these reasons, too, a layman's guide to treatments can only be a general outline. But it does help the patient and family to know what is helpful—or not helpful—in any given condition, and to have an idea of what is available.

For instance, preparations come in a variety of forms and some may suit one person and not another. Lotions are usually prescribed for scalp treatments because they are simple to apply, although for severe psoriasis or eczema of the scalp it may be necessary to use a cream, jelly or ointment which is afterwards washed out with shampoo.

The choice between a cream and an ointment is often simply a matter of personal preference, though one may suit a certain type of skin more than another. Ointments are greasier and usually better for a very dry condition, whereas creams penetrate the skin easily and may therefore be more effective on a greasy skin, and more suitable cosmetically.

Some preparations contain lanolin, preservatives, perfume or an ingredient such as an antibiotic which the user finds irritating or to which he or she is allergic. It is therefore always important to make sure that if a rash gets worse this isn't because of the ointment or cream being applied. This should usually be obvious, since the rash will be aggravated soon after application.

It is also possible for the skin to become so used to a particular preparation after long-term use that it stops being effective, so it may be time to ring the changes for a while. Eventually the original ointment or cream may help again.

Treatments for skin conditions will also involve a choice between the *topical* and the *systemic*. The term topical describes the creams, ointments and lotions applied to the outside surface of the skin. Systemic remedies are tablets taken by mouth, or drugs injected straight into the blood stream. In particularly serious cases, steroids are administered short-term this way for adults.

A few fairly recent discoveries are revolutionising the treatment of certain skin conditions. But the older forms of care still have a place, and for both psoriasis and eczema various mixtures of coal tar are still used in creams, pastes and impregnated bandages.

Quite why coal tar has this healing effect on skin disorders is not known, but it certainly has soothing properties, relieves irritation and removes scales. Zinc oxide is another old-fashioned preparation still in use, and dithranol is widely prescribed for psoriasis. There can also be enormous help from various simple balms, oils and lubricating and moisturising creams to keep the skin soft and to reduce scaling.

Some psoriasis patients have regular treatment with ultra-violet B lamps to simulate sunlight, either alone or with tars or dithranol. Photochemotherapy—or PUVA as it is known for short—involves exposure to ultra-violet A light two hours after taking psoralen tablets to make the patient more sensitive to the rays. But this can be used only under strict medical supervision, and for severe cases, as the long-term side effects are still not known. In the same way the cytotoxic drugs which inhibit cell division and have had such a dramatic effect in some cases of psoriasis are not widely in use because they are toxic and side effects are still uncertain.

Special baths are also a regular part of treatment for various skin conditions. For psoriasis these baths contain tar, and for eczema emulsifying ointment or oil replaces soap, lubricating the skin and replacing lost oils. Oatmeal can also be a helpful old-fashioned remedy, as it helps to maintain the water content of the skin and is very soothing. Potassium permanganate soaks are another traditional remedy still in use, particularly helpful when eczema affects the soles of the feet.

The irritation caused by several skin disorders, including eczema, is helped by the use of antihistamines taken in tablet and syrup form, usually at night but also during the day. Because the skin is sensitive it also helps to wear cotton next to the skin rather than wool or nylon, and to avoid irritant substances such as feathers in pillows and duvets.

Dust is another irritant best kept at bay, for here something of a vicious circle exists. Dust mites feed off skin scales, and since patients with some disorders tend to have dry skins and lose these scales frequently, the mites have a field day. So it is important in treatment to keep the house, and particularly the bedroom, as dust-free as possible. Diet is also worth looking into—but more about this in Chapter 5.

Where eczema appears to be of the contact form in an adult, skin tests can be carried out by a dermatologist in the out-patient department of a hospital. This is a simple process and different from the prick testing for asthma when extracts from various substances actually enter the blood stream. In patch testing substances are held in contact with the skin for a length of time, and if a redness or rash appears in that area the allergy may be traced.

However, patch testing is not always reliable on its own, and must be done in conjunction with close questioning on the patient's lifestyle and observation of other factors. A rash which comes up persistently when a person comes in contact with a particular substance at work, or when wearing some item of clothing or jewellery, may indicate contact eczema. Eliminate the substance, and with any luck the rash will disappear.

There have also been important steps forward in the treatment of acne over recent years, particularly abroad, and even in a teenager it is certainly no longer something that people should be told to simply "sit back and live with".

Even so, the acne patient tends to rely on self-medication more than most. This may be partly because of the number of proprietary products on the market claiming miracle cures, and partly because of the fear that going to the doctor is making too much of a trivial complaint. Even when acne afflicts older people to a serious degree, they can carry on for years thinking it is not the sort of ailment to take to their G.P.

Yet there have been major breakthroughs both in the treatment of acne and in understanding its causes. Basically the treatments revolve round unblocking the pores, reducing the production of sebum in the body, controlling any infection and minimising the resulting inflammation. The first can be done by the use of various lotions and creams containing substances such as benzoyl peroxide which has a peeling effect. Patients with more severe acne will also need to take tablets to control both sebum and bacteria. The most commonly used are called tetracyclines.

Because of acne's connections with hormone imbalance, it has also been found that some women patients are helped by taking certain types of contraceptive pill, and in later years a course of oestrogen. It may be in this area of hormone control that further breakthroughs in treatment could occur. Also, interesting trials are taking place at present in this country using a form of chemically produced Vitamin A which dramatically cuts down the production of sebum. There is more about this in the research section of the last chapter.

Rosacea is also treated with antibiotics. Here is, however, a very good example of the slight but crucial differences between one skin disorder and another. Though spots may look like acne, the flush of rosacea does not and there are subtle differences in treatment. For some time steroids were thought to improve the condition and then it was found that by thinning the skin they were actually making the flush worse.

Another example of the importance of correct diagnosis is the similarity between urticaria and eczema. Urticaria should not be treated with steroid creams and ointments. Eczema, on the other hand, should not be treated with the antihistamine in topical form that is so helpful to the type of urticaria which follows a wasp sting or some other localised reaction. Antihistamine taken orally is prescribed for both conditions, however. It is precisely because of all these contradictions and complications in treatment that medical guidance is needed, plus a good working knowledge of treatment in patients themselves. Without adequate awareness it would be so easy to apply the wrong treatment to the wrong condition.

With some of the rarer conditions there is little that can be done other than ease the discomfort. In others it may be necessary simply to resort to cosmetic disguise until improvement occurs; people with alopecia can wear a wig, for instance, while waiting for the hair to grow back again. Certain forms of surgery can be used on birth marks including the revolutionary laser ray treatment mentioned in our research section, although all birthmarks need careful examination before any action is taken. Some of the strawberry marks disappear spontaneously anyway, and camouflage in the form of a good masking cream may be all that is necessary.

In certain of the more serious skin conditions and in severe cases of more common ones such as psoriasis, eczema and acne, treatment may be prescribed or given in hospital, either as inpatient or outpatient. Anyone with a persistent rash who would like a second opinion has every right to ask the GP for an appointment with the local skin specialist.

Some people with chronic conditions regularly spend periods in hospital, finding that the bed rest, the freedom from everyday pressures and responsibilities, the sterile atmosphere and regular medication all help in clearing the condition up. Even though the problem may return, at least they are making a fresh start and have had some respite from the usual discomfort.

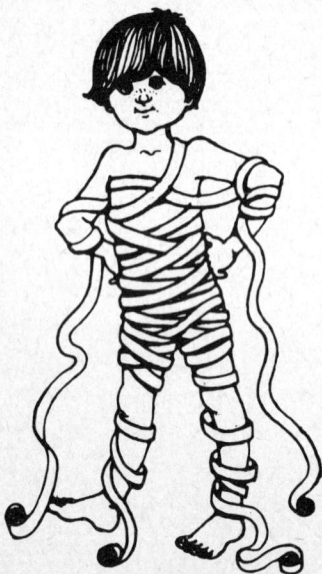

Treatment is best carried out in the evening when there is less pressure on time

Treating Yourself

But having received diagnosis and suitable suggestions for treatment, it is usually up to the patients themselves to put their regime into daily action. Armed with lotions and creams, tablets and potions it is for them to see that treatment is carried out as prescribed.

For many a chronic skin condition to cope with means application of the treatment day in and day out—which is its own problem. The treatments are usually long-term, and such that if discontinued the symptoms will return. To keep up the creaming and bathing and tablet-taking indefinitely is time consuming and tedious, and often strategically difficult, if for instance the patient is away from home.

On top of this, many of the more old-fashioned treatments are cosmetically unsatisfactory, and even the newer creams take time to apply and leave the skin looking greasy and shiny. All this can add to a person somehow feeling different or even untouchable.

In the book *Medieval Encounters*, Ray Jobling describes his daily ritual at one period as follows:

"Coal tar had been replaced by dithranol, which is as sticky and messy as the former, smells only slightly less strongly but is if anything even less acceptable to the patient in view of its affect of irritating and staining dark brown the as yet unaffected areas of skin adjacent to the psoriatic lesions."

He goes on to detail the considerable work involved in the shape of daily, lengthy soaking in tar baths; daily one or two-hour-long applications of unpleasant ointments; once or twice weekly attendance for ultra-violet treatment and four-to-six weekly visits to dermatological clinics. Much of this, he found, involved extra work for others, particularly his parents.

"The treatment demanded help from others in the application of ointments. Clothes and linen were constantly stained and spoiled, creating exceptional laundry problems (and a threat to respectability, since they were permanently brown, to hang out to dry as 'clean clothes') while the ever-present falling scales generated extra housework. The problem had an economic dimension in prescription charges, replacement clothing, etc. All of this was additional to the work of social management.

"I smelled constantly and peculiarly of coal tar. I was regularly absent from school for a morning at a time to visit the outpatients' department. Even in mid-winter I displayed a rich golden, unnatural tan. On more than one occasion some classroom misdemeanour or schoolwork failing prompted sarcastic remarks from a teacher unaware of the facts, with reference to people who 'would be better off spending more time indoors at their books and less out of doors acquiring a suntan'."

A mother whose child has eczema finds that at least an hour is added to the bedtime preparations by the special bath with emulsifying ointment that her daughter must soak in for twenty minutes plus the application of various creams and protective bandaging for certain areas. Hair must also be regularly shampooed with special shampoo to keep the eczema and scaling on the scalp under control.

Later chapters will explain in more detail helpful measures to take in coping with the child at home and at school. But as far as treatment is concerned, it is important that enough time be allowed to carry out treatment in an unflurried and peaceful way.

This period can be used positively as a special time when the child can be given lots of attention, talked to, cuddled and played with. One mother describes how she used to play a game with her child in which the ointments she dabbed on were the army attacking the enemy—the child's spots. Smoothing cream on can, in fact, be soothing emotionally as well as physically as we will see in a later chapter.

Those soaking baths can actually be enjoyed if the child has a story read to him or her, or the adult can use the twenty minutes to relax and to enjoy the pleasant sensation that a warm, oily bath can bring to a sore skin. For the school-age child and for the adult, treatment is probably best carried out in the evening when there is less pressure on time and when, once creams have been applied, you can retire comfortably to bed.

Trial, without, one hopes, too much error, will help in finding the particular preparations that are most acceptable and suitable for each individual and his or her life-style. This can be like looking for a needle in a hay-stack when for psoriasis alone there are over one hundred and eighty medical treatments available, but it will be worth the effort in the long run.

One man with psoriasis found that grease aggravated his condition and wanted something that was cosmetically acceptable and de-odorised. He eventually found what he wanted through reading the medical magazine *The Lancet* and was able to ask his doctor to prescribe it. In fact most doctors will be guided by a patient's discoveries about suitable preparations, and should find such suggestions helpful in prescribing. If a particular cream has made you uncomfortable or simply done no good, it is much better to say so.

There are also particular strategies that can help in fitting treatments into daily life. A specialist describes in *Beyond the Ointment* how severe psoriasis on a man's scalp was brought under control by intensive daily treatment for a short length of time, which gradually tailed off as the condition improved. The simpler, more cosmetically attractive lotions were applied at rush-hour time in the morning; the heavier ointments in the evening, to be shampooed off either later that evening or early next morning. As the condition improved the treatments became less frequent and in the end he was using them only twice a week.

Some people find it does the skin good to take a rest from treatments every now and then, particularly if on holiday. Plain lubricating creams or emulsifying ointment can be used as an experiment, and if the rash returns or becomes worse, then the usual treatment can be restarted. Not only does this give the skin a rest, it can give the patient a break from the work of medication, too.

Cutting back periodically on treatment also makes sense

financially. Prescription charges are rising, and adults have to spend a great deal of money on the preparations they are prescribed. Unlike some other chronic conditions needing constant medication, such as epilepsy, skin conditions are not exempt under the NHS from prescription charges for adults under retiring age.

However, many patients find that Pre-payment Certificates, which are a type of season ticket for prescriptions, very useful. If you have to pay prescription charges regularly, you can limit the amount by making a single payment in advance. Certificates can be bought to cover six and twelve-month periods, and they entitle you to reduced prescription charges over that period. You can get a form at any Post Office which gives more details.

Side-effects of drugs are another aspect of treatment that gives many patients worry, particularly as most of the time they are themselves responsible for administering them. Says one mother: "The antihistamine my son has to have at night certainly eases the irritation and helps him sleep, but it also has the effect of making him drowsy in the morning. He can often hardly wake up and get himself to school, and even when he is there tends to feel drowsy and out of touch for much of the morning. Any further doses taken during the day will have the same results."

Similarly an adult who is regularly on antihistamine tablets finds that even the occasional drink is out of the question because the two don't mix. Nor is driving recommended because of the drowsiness and lack of co-ordination that anti-histamine can cause. This mother questions the advisability of being long-term on a drug such as this, just as some acne patients wonder whether they should use antibiotics for months on end, and eczema and psoriasis sufferers question whether they should use steroids at all.

Where self or family treatment is usual, as in skin conditions, it is essential that the patient and the family understand the long-term effects of the preparations and how to apply them properly. Luckily more doctors and specialists are realising the importance of this now, and are prepared to discuss the pros and cons of various treatments with patients.

In acne, for instance, success of treatment will hinge on continuing it consistently for at least six months, since response is often slow and the results cumulative. Sometimes there is a fast improvement followed by a relapse, and the patient needs to know that the answer is to persevere rather than give up at that stage. Later, when improvements are obvious, the drugs can be cut down, but increased again with safety if the acne makes any further comebacks.

Oral antihistamines, in spite of the sleepiness they can cause, are medically safe. One specialist says that since reactions to them are very individual it is worth experimenting with different types. For instance, in both liquid and tablet form there are some that take effect for as little as four hours and some for as long as twelve. He also recommends that the antihistamine be taken when possible at night, because it can affect co-ordination, and as well as making driving a little risky this might well influence a child's concentration at school or an adult's at work.

Some of the other treatments in use, such as PUVA for psoriasis, are at such an early stage that results must be monitored carefully. The same applies to the toxic drugs that can have great success in clearing psoriasis but whose side-effects long-term are still unknown.

Facts about Steroids

But perhaps the most controversial area over recent years has been the use of steroids for skin conditions. Newspaper headlines and rumours picked up from relatives and friends have scared some people off completely, and there is no doubt that on some occasions these preparations have been over-prescribed. Cases have come to light of people who have been made ill or even died through over-application of topical steroids, and the condition of many patients has probably been made worse by their excessive use.

One mother whose child has psoriasis writes: "Since she was tiny she has been prescribed a variety of steroid creams of various strengths, none of which has cleared up the condition.

The specialist I went to see earlier this year prescribed a course of stronger steroid creams, and these I used as directed. However the day after I finished the creams the psoriasis which still had not disappeared broke out in areas where it had never been before.

"When I returned and told this to the specialist he wasn't surprised and said this often happened. When I asked if these drugs could cure, he said they couldn't and the dosage would have to be increased as time went by."

The mother describes this particular specialist as abrupt, rude and intolerant of any suggestions. "When I said I couldn't see the point in continuing with further courses, now highly irritated he accused me of not caring enough for my child and declared that he could not sit back and watch one of his children suffer in the same way."

This story is disturbing on two counts. First because of this specialist's apparent lack of knowledge about strong steroid preparations which on the whole are not recommended long-term for use on babies and children, and no longer considered to be suitable for certain psoriasis when the rebound reaction described takes place.

But just as sad is the specialist's attitude to the mother whose worries were perfectly reasonable and who could have benefited so much from reasoned explanations and further discussion.

If patients are armed with the correct facts about steroid preparations and how to use them, these can be a great help, particularly in controlling eczema. Their use in psoriasis is being questioned at present because of the rebound effect, but even here in the milder adult cases, if properly monitored they will have their uses.

Because correct application and understanding is so important, the National Eczema Society have issued a leaflet written after consultation with medical advisers which spells out the facts. As the leaflet explains, steroid preparations are laboratory produced hormones which are similar to the cortisol produced naturally by the body to control inflammation. Applied to the skin, they have the same effect of controlling inflammation and reducing the rash and soreness. Hydrocortisone is simply cortisol which has been produced in a laboratory, and it is the weakest of the steroid preparations.

The large range of other preparations which come under a variety of names are specially formed to be more powerful, and may have other ingredients added, including lubricants and sometimes antibiotics. Though basically similar in make-up, some are far stronger than others, and it is important to know this if steroids are to be applied correctly. The leaflet lists the preparations in order of their strengths, since no indication is given on the tubes themselves.

The basic rule to remember when applying the preparations is to use as little as possible to keep the skin condition under reasonable control. This means that they should be restricted to once or twice a day, and rather than being applied thickly like face cream should go on in a smear so thin you can hardly see it. Particularly in the case of the very strongest, the steroid preparations are best used for limited periods and alternated with weaker hydrocortisone or alternatives such as coal tar or lubricating creams. On the sensitive skin of the face and groin only hydrocortisone should be used.

The main reactions of the skin after over-use are stretching and thinning and possible increased growth of hair. The stretching shows itself rather like the stretch mark of pregnancy, with creases on the skin and loss of elasticity. The thinning will reveal blood vessels through the skin, particularly on the face, and this can mean a rather ruddy complexion.

Other side-effects, the NES leaflet explains, are internal reactions of the body, and since a great deal of steroid has to be absorbed into the bloodstream for these to take place they are unlikely to result from the correct use of topical steroids but can happen after long use of systemic steroids.

However, the internal side effects can include swelling of the face (moon face as it is called), the slowing of growth in babies and children, and adrenal suppression which can lead to the body producing less natural cortisone, so that if the patient has a shock or operation there is less resistance to infection or trauma.

Something that many people are unaware of is that when systemic steroids are being given a special card should be issued to the patient and shown for at least two years after a course of treatment when other medical attention is required. Immunisation with live vaccine should also be avoided by those on systemic steroids, and this includes polio, measles and yellow fever. In fact one specialist's advice is always to mention steroid treatment of any sort when attending a clinic for injections.

When on repeat prescriptions it is necessary to see the doctor every few months, so that he or she can keep an eye on the skin's progress. Even if a patient decided to come off steroid preparations for a time, this should never be done overnight as the rebound effect already mentioned will take place and the rash may become even worse. Instead, tail off gradually, introducing a new treatment over a period of a week or so or even longer.

It is encouraging to hear that research is continually going on in the drug manufacturing companies and hospitals into safer methods of treatment, and that when a new formula is produced there should be many trials and studies before it is finally launched for public use.

It must, for instance, meet with the approval of the Committee on Safety of Medicines, a body set up as a watch dog for the public interest. Manufacturers also have their own watch dogs, the Association of the British Pharmaceutical Industry, which has a Code of Practice covering the marketing and promotion of prescription medicines and which represents manufacturers who supply ninety-nine percent of sales to the National Health Service.

Dermatologists also work with these drug companies, and teams of researchers and laboratory technicians are continually on the look-out for new breakthroughs in treatment. I suppose that we all hope for the miracle preparations that will actually cure all skin conditions rather than simply suppress the symptoms. But for the moment, if a person is at least helped to face the world it makes life a good deal better for them.

One mother of a seven-year-old boy with chronic eczema

stopped using steroids for a year because of her worries about side-effects. During that year he spent eight weeks in hospital in the hot summer months bandaged from head to foot in an effort to clear his skin with more old-fashioned methods. As the year went on and the eczema became worse he became increasingly uncomfortable, unable to play football or even walk at times because his skin was so dry and sore.

"In the end we had to make the choice between using steroids again and allowing him to lead a normal life, or continuing without them while we watched him turn into an unhappy semi-invalid. After a year of struggle we chose the first course and now he is leading a very full life again, appearing in school plays and playing his beloved football.

"We do, however, use the steroid preparations as sparingly as possible and ring the changes from time to time, trying to keep to the weaker hydrocortisone and only working our way up the ladder to the stronger steroids when the rash is really bad."

Another eczema sufferer, this time an adult, describes how she stopped using steroid creams on her face and finds she can get by with ordinary lubricating lotion instead. But she still feels there is much to be said for steroid treatments if they help, even short courses of those taken orally.

"I first went out with a boyfriend when I was eighteen when I had been on steroids about nine months. They helped to clear up my skin, they gave me a normal young person's life, they gave me boyfriends and later I went to Australia and met my husband there.

"But before I was on steroids my skin was still very bad and I would not go out and mix with people. So I do feel that in severe cases of eczema, which mine was, that steroids should be considered. Yes, I know that I have stretch marks on the inside of my thighs and a little on my legs, but people don't see them, they don't stare and I wear bikinis happily on the beach."

Sometimes talking with other patients or attending a talk at a group meeting, or even reading a medical magazine like the psoriasis patient quoted earlier, people will hit upon a treatment they have never heard of before. One mother, for instance, heard for the first time the correct way to melt emulsifying ointment in boiling water before adding it to the nightly bath. For another mother this bath carried out twice a day actually cleared her child's condition.

A psoriasis patient describes in *Beyond the Ointment* his own four-point plan for treatment, which started with avoiding the factors he found seemed to make him worse, such as hot baths, stress, central heating and alcohol in excess. Lesson two was to find the treatment and frequency that holds the skin condition within acceptable limits and stay with that.

"I found that the essential treatment consisted of removal of the scales without damage or irritation of the surrounding and underlying skin. I discovered which treatments did this most satisfactorily, and I found that the appearance of the lesions became more acceptable at the same time. At certain times when my psoriasis became bad, I found that I could arrest it by intensive treatment and similarly at other times I found that I didn't have to bother.

"I also found that my psoriasis tended to oscillate and that to complete a cure would result in a subsequent recession, and that it was, therefore, much more acceptable to find an intermediate position and avoid this morale-destroying up and down."

So lesson three was to find the middle course. His fourth lesson was to recognise the skin condition in yourself and treat it appropriately.

"Too greasy an ointment required too much cleansing and the skin could become over-dry. Alternatively a vanishing cream base might in itself be too drying. So I learned to recognise my skin condition and to apply lotion, cream or ointment as appropriate. Similarly I found a shampoo that was not too harsh nor too mild."

A woman with acne describes how throughout her teenage years and into her twenties she put up with her chronic acne, always thinking that it might go away but finding that none of the proprietary brands of preparations that she bought from chemist shops did any good.

"Then I tried a new treatment from the doctor, and after persevering for some time the acne improved tremendously. The difference this made to my life was amazing. For a start I felt so much more comfortable because the spots had been on my face and neck and they used to make me feel so stiff and sore. I also had some eczema on my hands, and this went away, too. I was able to start leading a normal social life again.

"I'm so glad now that I kept on with the treatment. I'd say to anyone with acne, especially teenagers, don't give up. You can be made better."

In his book *Skin Care*, Dr. Bethel Solomon, a skin specialist, underlines this fact.

"The rate of cure with carefully selected forms of treatment can be ninety percent and the remainder can be immensely improved," he says. "The worst statement that can be uttered to someone afflicted with acne is that nothing can be done about it and that time (spent in doing nothing) will lead to its gradual disappearance. It will gradually disappear, but in the meantime misery, frustration and self-consciousness will build up to an alarming degree."

His words echo what could safely be said about most other skin conditions. If it sends a teenager happily to a party or a mother contentedly out with her pram or means a good night's sleep for the whole family, then the trouble of treatment is worth the effort.

3 — Facing the World

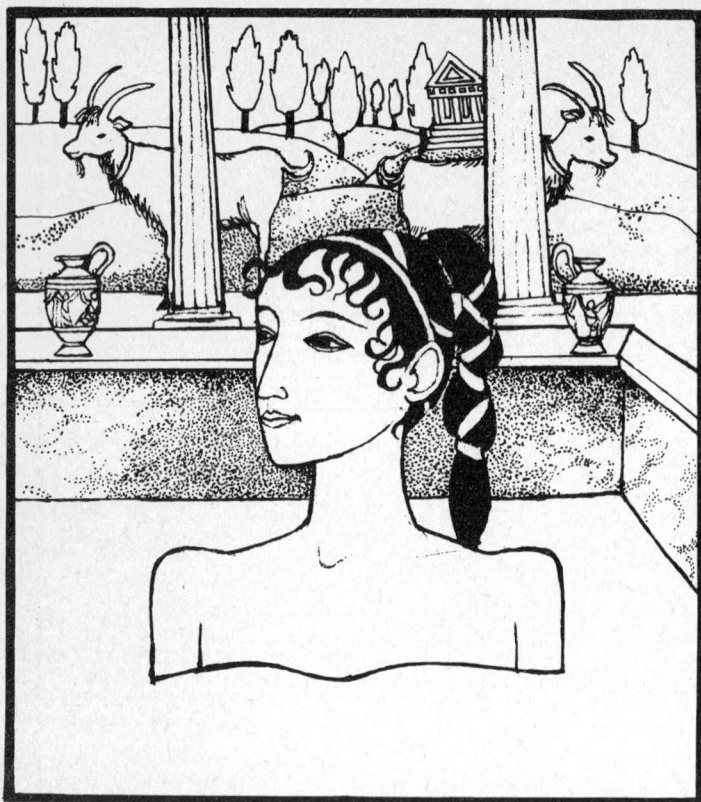

From the earliest times when goddesses bathed in milk the skin
has been a signal of beauty and attraction

"It is on my face and neck, and I look awful and feel like a
leper. I just can't bear to mix with people, and I am getting
more and more depressed. Although my doctor says the
treatment he is giving me will eventually clear it up, it's hard
to believe him. I feel quite alone and helpless because
nobody understands."   *Mary, aged 18*

"She won't stop scratching until she bleeds and then of
course we have the tears and the tantrums trying to clean

Becky and bandage her up . . . We do find shopping a problem with her. Unfortunately other parents don't understand and just tend to pull their children away thinking she's got some contagious disease.''   *Mother of Becky, aged 4*

''I've always tried hard not to be self-pitying and a moaner. But unless you've got it, you really can't understand what it's like. My skin peels off, literally, and my poor husband's practically beside himself seeing me like that and not being able to do anything to help.''   *Elsie, aged 42*

T HE three people quoted above all have one thing in common — they suffer from a skin disorder. In Mary's case it is acne, in Beckys it is eczema and in Elsie's it is psoriasis.

Though on the surface at any rate the conditions are all different, the underlying emotional and social problems these cause are very similar and typical of those suffered by most patients to some degree or other.

In Mary's case there is the worry that treatment just isn't doing any good and that her skin is never going to get better. She feels she is an outcast, disliked by everyone because her spots spoil her appearance, and she is becoming more and more isolated as she withdraws into herself.

In Becky's case there is the physical discomfort of an itchy, sore skin; the messy treatments; the emotional upset that all this causes a young child. For the parents there is the sadness of watching her suffering, the anxiety over carrying out some of the most ordinary everyday tasks of life, such as shopping, and the fears that other people think her rash is catching.

For Elsie there is the constant struggle to look on the bright side and not to let her problems dominate her life. But the sheer discomfort, the sometimes embarrassing messiness of it all and the effect her skin disorder can have on those closest to her just wears Elsie down.

And in every case there is mention of feeling that ''nobody understands''. Above everything else it is lack of understanding that can lead to the greatest distress for those with a skin disorder and those who live with them.

Yet it is this very understanding, both in the patient and in other people, that can be the key to learning successfully to live with the condition. As we've already seen, it is possible to find out why the skin itches or flakes, to discover the treatments and treatment routines which suit you best and to seek out correct information about the side-effects of various drugs. All this makes a great difference in coping with physical symptoms.

In the same way it is also possible to understand and deal with the social and emotional effects of these symptoms. Sometimes the answers may be purely practical, sometimes they may involve a change in attitude on the part of the patient or the family, and sometimes they require a change of attitude in others. But the answers are usually there in the end.

The trouble is, we often don't know where to look, so in some ways it is not surprising that patients, their families and the outside world find the problems connected with a skin condition hard to understand. In spite of new treatments and continuing research, doctors admit that for the moment some of the basic reasons behind skin disorders remain a mystery, and that though treatments may minimise symptoms they will not always control them entirely.

Old wives' tales still abound, and though the patient may be given lots of advice about day-to-day coping by well meaning neighbours and friends, it can be difficult to find accurate information. Doctors and specialists may be able to diagnose the rash and give prescriptions where necessary, but there often will not be time (or maybe inclination) to discuss with a mother whether or not she should wash her baby's nappies in detergent, or with a teenager how to improve his social life.

On top of this, the patient may often have to deal with lack of understanding in other people. Many whose skin is un-blemished simply don't want to know about those who itch and break out in spots and rashes—until it hits them, anyway. Though over ninety percent of the population go to their GP over skin rashes at some time in their lives, for reasons that probably go back centuries and are lost in the mists of folk-lore, skin disease is often seen as somehow unpleasant and taboo.

"We can be a cruel race. See someone with an erupting skin and we immediately flinch, take one step back," writes a newspaper columnist after a visit to the dermatology department of a large hospital.

"We wash our hands carefully as soon as we are able, for fear we've caught something. Kids at school won't hold hands with a child whose hands are affected. Some teachers have been known to ask mums to take their children home. Skin sufferers cover up what they can. What they can't they hide, at home, behind closed doors, fearing even the postman and milkman calling with milk bill or parcel."

Yet at the same time, side by side with this fear of skin disorders, one gets the impression that many people, even some of the medical profession, consider that they are almost trivial. To worry about them blows them out of proportion, rather like going on and on about the trials and tribulations of the common cold, annoying though this may be. Indeed, some might question whether the problems are there at all and are not simply the product of a few rather neurotic people's lively imaginations.

It's true that on the whole most skin conditions neither cripple in the physical sense nor kill. Yet it is also true that emotionally and socially they can cripple a person's life, and that in certain extreme cases this has led patients to kill themselves.

How people cope depends a great deal on the type and severity of the condition, of course. Skin disorders can vary enormously in degree, fluctuating from month to month and often clearing naturally as suddenly as they came. Whereas one person may be covered in patches of psoriasis or the rash of eczema, another will only have small areas. Whereas in one adolescent acne can arrive one week and be gone in six months time, in another it may linger on for years.

A lot will also depend on a person's natural temperament: the level of emotional upset over a skin disorder is not always clearly linked with its severity. A social worker attached to a large London hospital specialising in skin disorders says that how much these affect people depends quite often on personality and attitude. She cites the example of one man with both psoriasis and acne who, although at times socially embarrassed by his appearance, nevertheless enjoys a very happy marriage with three children and a good job. Because of his naturally confident disposition he can cope with his difficulties.

Yet think about it, and we all know how even a boil on the chin can affect our pride in ourselves, or the itch from a single gnat bite drive us practically mad at night. So it doesn't take much more thought to realise that even if a rash is mild or a condition relatively transitory it can still take its toll. How much worse this would be, then, if the condition were severe and lasted for years.

Fortunately more and more doctors are realising that the emotional and social effects of skin conditions can be as difficult to deal with as the physical ones, and are helping to do something about this.

Two specialists, one of whom is the founder of The Psoriasis Association, write in the *British Journal of Dermatology*: "There is a need to delineate where and when skin disease is interfering with normal living and to encourage self and community care so that some of the relevant load is taken away from established services."

Comments another dermatologist: "People with severe facial eczema, acne or psoriasis usually do not feel ill, they continue at work or school and often do not seek medical advice. Nevertheless the social and economic cost of 'silent' skin disease must be enormous." And says another: "To have a skin disorder can have a devastating effect—and it's not just vanity. It goes much deeper than that."

Dr Terence Ryan, who wrote the forward to this book, said at a conference on skin disorders held by the Disabled Living Foundation: "Consider a little girl born with a severe birth mark, an aversive handicap (i.e. one that is defined as unwelcome or unsightly). One has to take into account not only her life, the whole of her life, but the life of her family, her parents and the other children in the family. Its management calls at an early stage for the planning of her whole life.

"Especial sensitivity to injury from environment is illustrated by the child whose severe sensitivity to the sun resulted in disfigurement and virtual exclusion from society in normal daylight. I know of schoolboys who in any normal house or school in the winter develop severe damage from the cold—their schools merely find it inconvenient and are not particularly sympathetic, and so every winter at school they continue to develop severe destruction of the skin.

"There are patients who have an intolerable smell, others who suffer always from drenching sweat; how can such persons with aversive handicap be employed? These are not disorders which can be managed merely by a prescription, they require the co-operation of families, school teachers and employers. I keep going back to the problem of handicap—skin disease is a handicap."

One family doctor who has taken a particular interest in skin conditions and regularly treats patients with acne, psoriasis and eczema, also sees daily the sort of emotional and social problems from which they suffer.

"Skin disorders affect so many areas of people's lives, even to dictating what they wear," he observes. "Acne, for instance, can spread to arms, back and chest as well as face, and psoriasis can cover people in angry red patches with silvery scales which are shed all the time. People find this embarrassing. Women will wear trousers and long sleeves and try to cover the rash in make-up, even though this may aggravate the skin and on the whole a rash is best left uncovered.

"I see middle-aged women with acne, and at the moment I see a six-year-old child who has psoriasis. She is very bothered by this at school and her parents feel guilty because it is an inherited condition. Though I try to explain to parents they must not blame themselves, they often can't help it.

"Another major problem in conditions such as eczema, psoriasis and acne is the thought in others that what you have might be infectious and there is a need to reassure patients that their disorder is not contagious—they can't give it to anyone else. No doubt this fear stems from the fact that spotty illnesses like measles and chickenpox are infectious, as are certain skin conditions such as warts and impetigo. But the majority of long-term skin disorders including eczema, psoriasis and acne are not".

"Treatments can in themselves be messy and unpleasant. Thick smelly creams and flowery dresses don't really go together and often the nicer, more refined preparations aren't so effective. Another obvious disadvantage is that the skin condition can so easily be seen. The skin is the only organ of the body where progress—or lack of it— in an illness can be seen at work. If improvement is slow then this can have a disheartening effect on the patient since he is only too aware of the fact."

But perhaps the people who can explain the problems best are the patients themselves. In recent years, since the formation of numerous self-help groups, hundreds and thousands of letters and articles have recorded the patients' point of view.

Writes one woman who not only has chronic eczema herself but has three children with it as well: "I was born with it and asthma, and was told how people looked away after looking in the pram. I was covered from head to foot always in bandages. All through school I always seemed to be hiding myself, it was awful. I never had the pleasure of bathing the children, my hands were always a mess. My husband bathed them, he had to and still does."

"At this time I am unemployed because of my skin," writes a young man. "I lost my job in a textile factory three weeks before Christmas and am being helped by my hospital social worker. The heat is a problem with me. I cannot work outdoors or in a warm or hot factory."

"I would like to ask how do other adult sufferers cope with preparing food?" asks a woman whose rash affects her hands. "I find it a constant struggle. My husband's very understanding, but I worry about outsiders, even our own close relatives. Do you let them push you out of the kitchen like a helpless child, or stand up to them and prepare the food the best way you can, dying inside because you think it makes them feel sick to eat it?"

"I was horrified to learn my daughter had this nightmare of a skin disease," says a mother. "For years she cried and scratched until I thought that I was going mad. I was so alone and couldn't cope. Mealtimes were a nightmare for all the family. Then when I was forty I had another little girl who was covered with dry, red angry skin when she was born, and eczema was diagnosed.''

Writes a woman with psoriasis: ''I could never try another hairdresser. Where I go they know me and understand my illness. Imagine trying somewhere new—they'd probably take one look at my scalp and run off screaming. I really looked after my skin, ate all the right food, loved pretty clothes. Now it's trousers and long sleeves to hide the mess. I couldn't think of wearing an evening dress—not that I ever feel like going out nowadays.''

And writes a man with psoriasis: ''From being a healthy, sports mad youngster, I slowly turned into a semi-recluse, avoiding all physical activity in public and trying to escape the taunting cruelty and total lack of understanding of my fellow pupils and teachers. A few attempts to play games and swim when covered with plaques convinced me that discretion was the better part of valour.''

Recently, a woman with acne asked to hear of other patients' experiences for research she was doing. She was inundated with letters which poured out problems.

Some of the more unusual skin conditions can be all-embracing in their effects, influencing a whole life style. One woman with vitiligo, which in her case affects her entire body, describes how during the summer months when the normal areas of skin become tanned, the other areas remain white or burn to a bright lobster colour. The condition particularly affects her face which means she has to try to avoid all exposure to the sun.

Another patient suffers from light sensitivity, which means she comes out in a rash when exposed to the sun. ''The irritation can be so intense I hardly know what to do with myself. I used to hold my hands and arms under the cold water tap until they went numb. I remember bandaging my feet in cold tea to try and ease the agony.''

But quite apart from the physical discomfort, there are the practical aspects. To protect her skin from the sun she started wearing slacks for the first time in her life at a period when not many women dressed like this.

"With men's socks and thick shoes I was safe from the waist down. I found there was not sufficient protection in a long-sleeved blouse so however hot it was I always wore a jacket or cardigan as well. I used to keep my hair long all summer to protect my neck."

Finding the Answers

Such difficulties stemming from the physical symptoms of any given skin condition are typical, affecting all those involved with skin disorders, from the parent of the child with eczema who scours the shops to find cotton socks and tights to wear next to the skin, to the psoriasis patient who may spend hours experimenting with various shampoos to treat an affected scalp.

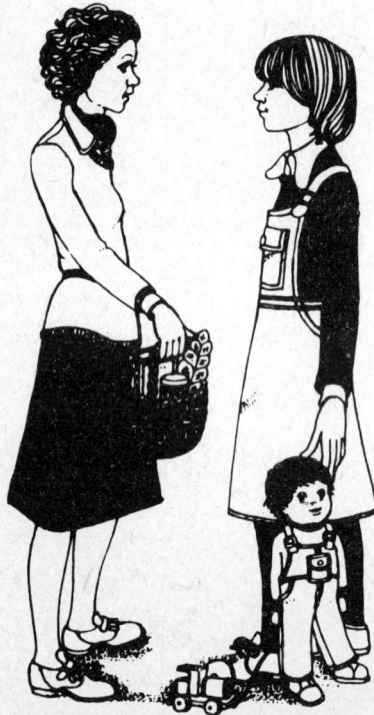

It can bring great comfort to talk to someone in the same situation

One young woman with eczema describes how she feels she can't go away for weekends because treatments make a mess on baths and bedclothes. Several times she has had to postpone her wedding because outbreaks landed her in hospital. Her working life became disrupted and her earnings reduced. On one occasion she was told by the labour exchange: ''Well, nobody will employ you with hands like that.''

But having posed some of the problems affecting people's lives, it is important to remember that the majority of situations are in the end resolvable and that even most of the case histories quoted here have happy endings. This young woman, for instance, did eventually get married and started work as nanny to a doctor's family.

The young man having trouble with employment benefited from a spell in hospital and his condition improved so that he could get back to everyday living again.

After making contact with another patient through a self-help group, the woman who was worried about preparing food because of her sore hands realised that she wasn't the only one to feel like this and received several encouraging tips. For instance, one fellow sufferer suggested wearing cotton-lined rubber gloves, not just for the sake of other people but because it was far more comfortable. ''I even eat my snack meals with them on when I am on my own, to avoid getting my hands sticky and having to wash them,'' she says. ''The improvement in my hands is incredible and my peace of mind bliss.''

The two mothers quoted above found that simply writing about their problems helped. ''I feel better for writing this down, it's just like talking to someone,'' says the first. ''It brings me much comfort to know there are so many parents in the same situation with the same problems to face. I didn't know this, but now I cope much better with my child than I did before,'' says the second.

A change in attitude—often so much easier to achieve once you have talked problems over or found some practical answer—may not spirit difficulties away overnight, but it will make them seem easier to cope with. I know from our own experience that though our son's condition has not changed very much over the years, our attitude to it certainly has. This has been mainly through our increased knowledge and understanding: treatments are now just a part of daily life and problems dealt with as they arise.

The man quoted earlier who found his psoriasis such a handicap in his youth still has the condition as an adult. But at a certain point he made up his mind to bring about certain changes both in his life style and in his psychological stance, so that now it is no longer the burden that it was. He feels in control of the disorder rather than controlled by it, and has a successful career and home life.

But perhaps what most people with a skin condition find hardest to come to terms with, is the feeling that they have been stigmatised and rejected. This is illustrated in many of the experiences quoted. It is important to face this problem, and to ask oneself first whether the stigma does really exist. There are times when it may simply be in the imagination of the person with the skin disorder.

"Yes, I do feel there is a stigma attached to this disease," says a woman with psoriasis whose face is affected as well as her body. "People cannot or will not try to understand it. Their initial reaction can be quite hostile—perhaps they think they might catch it, but it makes one's day-to-day life difficult.

"I have experienced a number of problems regarding this. On one occasion I was travelling on a bus and a woman came and sat down beside me, then turned, looked at me and said loudly: 'God, she's got rabies or something.' Whilst this may sound comical in retrospect, at the time I wished I could just melt into the background. What I did was get off the bus at the next stop."

And says the mother of three children with eczema: "You're cut to pieces watching someone who doesn't understand it take her children away from mine in case they catch anything. Or hearing my own children asking what they should say to children at school who want to know what their spots are.

"It affects your personality because you can't be yourself. You're forever making excuses people can't understand and it's most frustrating. I can't wear gloves all the time and when it is noticed people turn up their noses and pull away rather than touch your hand when handing something over.''

Power of Appearance

The power of the skin's appearance to attract or repel has always been with us. From the earliest times, when goddesses bathed in goat's milk, Egyptians painted their eyelids and Roman matrons dyed the palms of their hands with henna and used barley water and butter as a face cream, the skin has been the outward signal of beauty and attraction.

Nowadays, however much we would like to achieve a calm, unruffled attitude to a skin problem, films, magazines, newspapers, television and the rest of the media seduce our senses—or assault them—with the apparently over-riding necessity for a smooth and lovely skin from top to toe. As once cleanliness was thought to be next to Godliness, now it would seem to be an immaculate skin.

Articles and advertisements recommend this treatment and that preparation to achieve ultimate perfection, and beautiful people gaze reproachfully at us from photographs and roadside hoardings. Sometimes the skin is used to sell the most unlikely products. ''Perfect, pure simplicity'' croons one TV advertisement for a digital watch as the camera lingers in close-up on somebody's velvety bare limbs. ''Smooth line, uninterrupted by a single flaw.''

In his book *More Than Skin Deep*, American dermatologist Thomas Sternberg describes the role of beauty in the practice of dermatology as of utmost importance not only because to look one's best is mentally uplifting, imparts confidence, contributes towards our relationship with other people and our adaptation to the world, but also because to look unbeautiful is depressing, discouraging, and tends to lead to isolation and withdrawal?

In his opinion patients often go to the dermatologist as much to improve their appearance as to rid themselves of an ailment. He cites the example of a forty-five year old woman patient who had aged so much and become so depressed that she had taken to drink.

But even worse, he says, is the situation of the young girl who must meet the world with her confidence completely shattered by a severe acne with pits and postules, or of the psoriasis patient who wakes up each morning in a bed "full of scales but otherwise empty".

Quite apart from appearance, some of the reasons why there should be any stigma attached to skin disorders are more obvious than others. As a GP has already pointed out, unlike a stomach ulcer or weak kidney where the ailment remains hidden, a rash or blemish on the skin can be easily seen. The patient is continually reminded of it, as are those who look at him or her.

Then there is the fear that all skin conditions are infectious. As the same GP has explained, though this may be based on misconceptions and the muddling of one disorder with another, it is extremely difficult to convince every member of the public that this is so. Many people, some patients included, still think that you can pick eczema up in a train or catch psoriasis or acne from sharing a towel.

The connection of skin disease with neglect, dirt and lack of hygiene is equally unjustified these days, though in days gone by there were indeed terrible diseases caused through poor sanitation, squalid surroundings, inadequate diet and lack of suitable treatments. In the Bible people to be healed from skin disorders were told to "go and get clean", so that even today the word "clean" is sometimes used to describe a blemish-free skin.

Until fairly recently many dermatologists were also concerned with the treatment of venereal disease, and one specialist feels that even if it is only at a subconscious level people may still equate skin disorders in general with venereal infections, infusing them with the same uncleanness and shame commonly associated with such complaints. Then again there are old associations with the dreaded leprosy, even when the leper himself is no longer shunned as once he was.

Certain symptoms could also have a part to play in suggesting to the uninformed that lack of hygiene may be a cause of skin disorders. For instance, a sore skin is more vulnerable to infection than one that is whole. The blocked pores of acne can be so far beneath the skin's surface that they are unreachable by washing, yet people still recommend a good scrub.

Treatments for eczema and psoriasis often do involve baths, but these are to allow preparations such as tar for healing and oil for lubricating to be more effective. Even some of the preparations used in treatment can create an illusion of grubbiness; tar pastes stain the skin brown and ointments give the skin a greasy look.

Once again we seem to come back to the need for better understanding. If more people realise the true facts about skin conditions and know for sure that they are not infectious, dirty or in some way self-generated, then perhaps they will be able to treat the patient and his family with more sympathy.

The same will go for the person with the skin disorder. The more he or she understands about a condition, the more easily she can explain it to other people, and cope with it day-to-day in a practical manner. Attitude will again make a lot of difference when dealing with feelings of rejection or stigma.

The majority of us are vulnerable to public opinion and find it hard to stand up to some obvious defect in our appearance. As one useful book—Erving Goffman's *Stigma: Notes on the Management of a Spoiled Identity*—points out, most people feel stigmatised in some way, whether from possessing a long nose, a small bust, or a criminal record! Also, what one person considers a stigma another may not.

The book discusses the possibility that for some the feeling of stigma can be used as an excuse for every bit of bad luck that comes along. A scarred face, for instance, could become the hook on which the patient has hung all his inadequacies, all his dissatisfactions, all his procrastinations and failings in life: he has come to depend on it not only as a reasonable escape from competition but as a protection from social responsibility.

But if the scar is removed by surgery, says the book, and the patient cast adrift from the more or less acceptable emotional protection it has offered, he soon finds that life is not all plain sailing even for those with unblemished "'ordinary' faces".

It is also possible to stigmatise ourselves, perhaps bringing our own prejudices to judging what other people think of us. Says one woman with acne: "I can quite understand people not wanting to come near me as I don't like spots either." Says a woman with eczema: "It is messy, unpleasant to the touch and the sufferer can leave behind her a trail of scabs, flakes of skin or even blood stains. We are unreasonable to expect sympathy and understanding from non-sufferers . . ."

From his experience the chairman of the Psoriasis Association, Ray Jobling, who is a sociologist and also a long-term sufferer from psoriasis, feels that as important as whether or not other people think of a skin condition as unpleasant or unsightly is whether or not the patient himself does so.

In one survey carried out by the Psoriasis Association, over eighty percent of the two hundred taking part mentioned effects on social contacts and relationships. More than one third specifically referred to embarrassment and self-consciousness, and over a quarter mentioned unsightliness and disfigurement. Many others complained of being stared at or questioned by strangers.

"Significantly, however, only a tiny majority had themselves actually experienced at first hand any clear act of avoidance or exclusion as a result of their skin condition," he points out in *Exchange*, the magazine of the National Eczema Society. "While no one would deny that unpleasant incidents occur, it is possible that these are more rare than might at first seem to be the case.

"Ignorance in relation to skin disease may be widespread, there may be misapprehensions or stigma. Certainly skin sufferers should press for research to clarify this position. But probably more important is the sufferer's belief that such a problem exists.

"In this sense the 'problem' may be the sufferer's own fearful anticipation of negative judgements and the nagging uncertainty about the impression that he is making as a result of the obtrusiveness of the skin disorder. Having daily examined oneself closely and possibly magnified the blemish to such an extent that it overwhelms all other features of one's person and personality, it is hard to accept that others are not acutely aware of one's skin condition, too.

"Constantly searching for an explanation or reason for our disorder, we cannot easily accept that others are just as likely to take it for granted as just another allergy, inherited tendency etc. as they are to attribute guilt and responsibility to us."

Again, this aspect was brought home to me by two incidents when I was researching this book. In one, a friend with whom I was discussing the fact that a mutual acquaintance had psoriasis and we had never realised it, said that he never looked at people's skins, just their eyes and features.

On another occasion, meeting some people for a drink, I saw that one had suddenly developed what seemed a very obvious rash on her face. When two of us left and I was wondering out loud why one never discussed a rash or spots in the way that one would enquire about a cough or a broken arm, my companion said: "What rash? I didn't notice."

As both a sufferer and a person with considerable experience of other people's problems, Ray Jobling suggests that the best way to cope socially is with openness, directness and simple straightforward explanations, then allowing other things to become the focus of attention. "On the other hand imperfect attempts to cover up and an embarrassed evasiveness may provoke suspicion or attract unwanted attention," he says.

One man tells the story of how he went to a crowded beach with a friend who had extensive psoriasis on his body. When the man was in his bathing suit they got the distinct impression that the area around them had cleared a little, but undeterred the pair of them took their swim and returned to the beach to dry off.

It was then that, one by one, far from going away, people started to draw closer. First one then another came up to discuss the psoriasis, confiding either that they had suffered from it themselves at one time or that they had a relation or friend who did. They asked questions about the disorder, compared knowledge and generally talked with an openness and friendliness that could never have been the case if the man had not had the honesty and bravery to take his swim.

One man who joined the Psoriasis Association and attended meetings found that he learned more in a few hours from listening to talks from a dermatologist and an informed layman than he had gleaned in twenty-five years. Reading the society's literature taught him even more.

"With a courage I had never known before, I went out into the world. I visited pubs, I enjoyed my most social Christmas for many years. I answered the quizzical looks at my skin with an attempted joke and a brief explanation, but often found I was only imagining that people saw me as something to be shunned or looked at with suspicion. I found an understanding barber whom I had never dared approach before.

"I started to live, and not only with my psoriasis. My increased knowledge gave me a new mental approach which was the answer to over half my personal battle. Is it just coincidence that I feel better than I have for years, that my dreaded itch is no longer so troublesome and indeed that the psoriasis has improved? I do not think so."

A change in public understanding where prejudice does exist can't happen overnight, but more publicity of the true facts about skin disorders, more general realisation of the physical, social and emotional problems involved and more available information and advice for the patient and his family will all help towards improvement.

As one man with eczema suggests: "Learn to understand the condition in yourself or your child. Learn to understand the lack of knowledge in others about skin disorders when it seems you are being mistreated or discriminated against—and, where possible, educate.

"Above all, learn to understand the limitation of your doctor or consultant. It is equally frustrating for him or her to see you suffer and the treatment fail sometimes. Notwithstanding my problems and setbacks, without the skilled aid of the medical profession I doubt if I would have achieved all that I have in education, career and marriage."

But this understanding process has to be two-way if incidents such as the treatment of the psoriasis patient on the bus quoted in this chapter are never to happen again. Says the woman concerned:

"As it is obvious that I am not going to be cured or get a remission in the foreseeable future I decided almost from the start not only to live with the thing but to try my hardest not to let it affect my life nor that of my family.

"All I ask is understanding—the understanding of my husband and sons I have, that of my work colleagues I think I have. I would like the general public to know of and try to understand the disease and to stop treating me and fellow sufferers like lepers."

4 – All in the Mind?

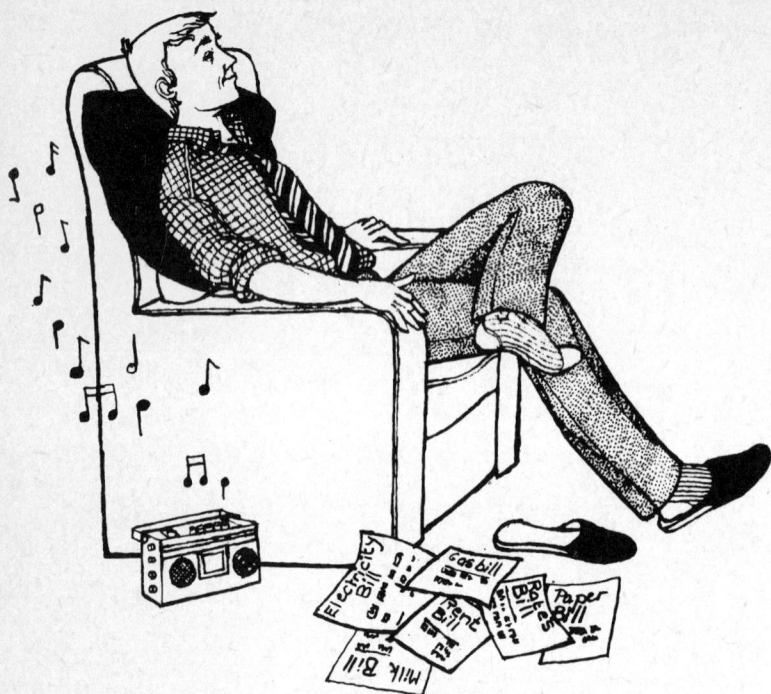

Some may find that a new interest such as music can help minimise the natural strains of life

"I'm not a nervous person or highly strung. I'm not under any stress. We have our own house and I'm very happily married."   *Eczema patient, aged 22*

"I cannot believe the cause of my daughter's psoriasis is emotional, as she has been quite seriously affected since she was very tiny. Also she is an extremely even-tempered little girl with a sunny disposition."   *Mother of Jane, aged three*

"My face felt so taut and painful, and every morning when I woke up there would be another spot. I was getting suicidal, just not wanting to wake up in the morning."

Acne patient, aged 42

MORE than most health problems, skin disorders tend to be put down to anxiety and stress—the outward and visible sign of an inwardly screwed up nature. "Oh, that's to do with nerves, isn't it?" people will ask, as if this neatly sums up the whole problem.

Yet one of the longest standing mysteries of all connected with skin conditions is their relationship with the emotions and the nervous system. There seems no doubt that stress can play a part at any rate in triggering certain conditions, and perhaps also in making them worse. Similarly it is clear that there is a relationship between the mind and the skin. The blush of guilt, the pallor from fear or anger, the perspiration from anxiety or mental effort, the tingling of the scalp when scared or excited, all point to this connection.

No doubt, too, the person with a chronic skin condition, or her parent, will often give the impression of being nervous and anxious, whether it's Susan the young woman quoted above whose face is breaking out in red, scaly patches; the mother whose little girl is covered from head to foot in psoriasis; or someone like Barbara who in middle age is still suffering the daily traumas of acne.

But rather like the chicken and the egg, it is important also to question which comes first. Does anxiety cause the skin disorders, or is it possible that it is the other way round? A skin which itches and continually erupts in sore places is enough to turn the most placid into worried, tense and perhaps deeply depressed people.

The experience of just three normal, confident people I know illustrates how badly even a mild disorder can affect personality and attitude. One told me how a boil on her nose kept her in the house for three weeks, so ashamed did she feel of her appearance. Another well balanced friend suffering from ringworm, a short-term and curable skin condition, took to wearing high-necked jumpers to conceal the red weals on her neck from the public gaze.

A third, with a patch of impetigo on her usually highly attractive and blemish-free face, raced to the outpatients' department of the local hospital at midnight, so panic-stricken was she that the rash was spreading all over her. If that's what a short lived experience of a skin disorder does to usually well integrated people, just think what months and perhaps years of the same could do.

The whole question of nervous connections with skin conditions has not been helped by outmoded theories which have found their way into books written over more recent years, some unfortunately still stocked on the shelves of reference and reading libraries.

It is generally accepted nowadays that stress can play a part in most illnesses, from heart trouble to ulcers and even cancer. When we think of stress in these cases we may list worries over the mortgage, coping with an over-demanding job and business account lunches, or a house move. We might even move into deeper areas such as depression after a bereavement or divorce, or perhaps the repression of negative feelings such as anger.

But move into the world of skin conditions, and because of superstitious and half-thought-through ideas from years ago that still linger on, stress seems to take on a very different meaning. According to some of these old and not so old books, people with skin conditions are mostly very neurotic indeed, their mental hang-ups ranging from mother deprivation to father fixation to scratching as a form of masturbation.

A few examples of skin conditions are obviously psychological in origin, such as the itching caused by a phobia about mites, or the raw areas of skin and bald patches that result when a person attacks his own body with his finger nails. Skin sufferers will also number among their ranks some naturally neurotic and depressed people, just as will any group with a medical problem. But these are not sound reasons on which to base sweeping generalisations.

One book, for instance, describing a study of women with pruritis in the genital area, suggests that the rash was due to sexual and other neurotic difficulties; that the patients had grown up with a sense of frustration and had been—or felt—rejected by their mothers; that their hatred of the mother had led to an undue attachment to the father, and that their behaviour as children had been morose, sullen or difficult.

Pages on urticaria, another intensely itchy condition, describe patients variously as "a fiery tempered man"; "a chronically disgruntled woman"; "a spinster aged 41 who had always borne a grudge against life because her mother favoured the patient's sister"; and "an engineer, aged twenty-five, an erratic, impulsive emotionally and psychosexually immature young man."

Another book, written around the same time, found that women with alopecia—dramatic loss of hair—could be described as neurotic, and as socially, emotionally and sexually inhibited. Later, hair loss in men is described as an unconcious abandonment of the symbol of masculine aggressiveness and in women, as an unconscious abandonment of the "crowning glory" as a defence against sexual temptations and unconscious incestuous impulses.

If a lot of this were not so dangerous, it would be funny. As if living in a surreal Monty Python world, the authors seem desperately to be seeking out symptoms and behaviour to fit their own pre-conceived- and often wild-ideas. One gets the strong feeling that whatever the character, background or personality of the unfortunate skin patient, he or she just couldn't win!

Another book written only twenty years ago offers as clues to a doctor or dermatologist for recognising an emotionally disturbed personality, the suggestions that the patient may be "questioning", demand "an immediate appointment", make frequent changes of appointment, display hesitancy, anxiety or flippancy, be "over-anxious or indifferent, talkative or reticent, preoccupied, apathetic, euphoric, dishevelled or inordinately tidy". At least the writer covered most of the options!

Nor apparently is the skin patient allowed a mind of his own. Another passage points out that the emotionally disturbed patient may not follow advice about treatment, and may complain about the treatment or the actions of previous physicians!

It would seem a good thing for all involved with skin disorders if these old books were swept off the library shelves, or at any rate issued only in conjunction with a more recently published medical work on the subject called *Psychophysiological Aspects of Skin Disease* by Professor F. A. Whitlock. The author, an Australian dermatologist and psychiatrist, knocks most of the skin and sex theories on the head in a most refreshing and logical manner.

Basically, he takes issue with them because they are not based on controlled studies comparing one set of people who have skin conditions with another set who have not and because "what we look for we inevitably find". Dealing with the point made in one of the books referred to above, that patients suffering from pruritis are likely to have unsatisfactory marriages and to have experienced unhappy childhoods, he comments that "one is bound to enquire how many women without pruritis vulvae have shared the same fate." And on the psychological theory of urticaria, he comments: "To state that two thirds of thirty-five patients suffering from urticaria suffered from lack of maternal affection in childhood is an empty observation unless one knows how many individuals in the general population also believe they suffered this misfortune."

He points to two main difficulties which influence the reliability of studies on the relationship between psychosexual history and skin disorder. First, most are in the nature of things retrospective: by the time a patient attends for treatment, months or even years may have passed since the initial symptoms. In such circumstances it is almost impossible to disentangle the present mental states from that before the skin condition made its first appearance.

"Secondly, the absence of controlled studies allowing for comparisons between groups of patients makes it impossible to estimate the specificity of many of the alleged frequencies of marital, family, sexual and other conflicts discovered in patients suffering from itching of all kinds, particularly anogenital itching.

"In members of the general public devoid of such symptoms not every marriage is harmonious, and even in these enlightened days sexual experience does not always come up to expectations. The frequency of such misfortunes in general is difficult to estimate, but it is surely essential to do so before concluding that similar situations in the lives of itching patients have a direct causal bearing on the skin symptoms.''

In similar vein, Dr Whitlock questions the validity of the ''mother rejection'' theory in infantile eczema, and quotes the example of one mother with three children mentioned in an earlier book who had expressed a fear of handling and fondling them lest she should inadvertently injure them.

''Although it is believed that lack of close physical contact with the mother 'causes' the atopic dermatitis, it seems odd that the other two children—presumably equally 'rejected'—did not develop the dermatoses.''

Dr. Whitlock's reflection echoes accurately the puzzlement of so many mothers when faced with the obviously clear skins of some of their children, and the sore, itching skin of the one child in whom they have apparently caused such severe damage.

With tongue again in cheek, Dr Whitlock mentions how a 1930 study reported that some patients, particularly young women complaining of acne, blushed when asked questions about their sexual lives. From this it was deduced that they were suffering from rosacea (whose symptoms are spots as well as a flushed appearance) although as he says

''The commonplace observation that most young women blush when questioned in this way would have made unbiased investigators pause before placing too much significance on the phenomenon.''

Reporting a further study of psoriasis patients, Dr Whitlock observes that in a study of over two thousand patients with psoriasis, forty percent said that their psoriasis appeared when they were worried, and thirty seven percent said it was worse if they worried. But as he points out, worry is a somewhat vague term and could include anything from concern about the weather to acute financial crisis.

"As such it appears to be part of the human lot and one might guess that an unselected sample of the population would record minor or major variations in chronic disorders when worries are in the forefront of their minds."

It is not that Dr Whitlock dismisses stress as a possible, even if not completely proved, cause, of certain skin conditions. But he rightly disputes the far-fetched and often offensive theories that propose stress as the sole cause, so that the patient with a skin disorder must necessarily be seen as neurotic, even mentally ill, and riddled with deep-seated hang-ups, many of them sexual.

A more balanced view would surely be the acceptance of the possibility that the normal stresses and strains of life may affect a skin condition in a predisposed person, just as they might cause migraine in another or stomach ulcers in someone else. Equally important, stress should be seen as just one of many possible factors causing or worsening a skin disorder along with many inherited tendencies, cell formation, skin type, allergy, faulty diet, injury, hormone imbalance and much more.

As Dr Bethel Solomons says in his book *Skin Care*, how simple it would be if it could safely be said that all skin disease had nervous causes! He quotes the case of a bank manager whose father and grandfather had been managers before him. He developed an itchy rash over the backs of his hands and on the back of his neck, which started soon after learning his son had failed his entry examination to the bank.

An interview with his son revealed that he had never really wanted to spend his life there, and had only attempted the examination to please his father. The dilemma was explained to his parents, he succeeded in entering the navy as a career, and his father's eczema responded to the change.

But as the author says, dozens of cases could be quoted of bank managers with obstinate sons or sons with dominating fathers working in banks who never had the slightest blemish on their skins. "This would quickly nullify what seemed to be an easy answer to the effect that emotional upsets have on the skin.''

It is unfortunate that even though some of the dustier cobwebs festooning skin conditions are at last being blown away, much of the damage is hard to put right. This shows its effects in the biased theories that many still hold, occasionally even in the medical profession, which tend to swing from one extreme to the other.

''I do feel annoyed by the attitude of those who attribute eczema to 'nerves', the implication being that willpower is the only cure required,'' says one patient. Says another; ''I was given the old line that 'it is because you are a woman. You will be alright when you marry and have children. It is all in your mind—an irritating skin shows an irritating nature!' ''

Conversely, the old theories have caused some dermatologists and doctors completely to dismiss the emotional aspects of skin disorders, whether as cause or effect. In his book *Essentials of Dermatology* Dr J. L. Burton comments:

"The role of psychological factors in causing or aggravating skin disease is controversial. Much nonsense has been written on this subject in the past, and this uncritical and uncontrolled work has produced a reaction among some dermatologists against psychosomatic concepts which may not be entirely justified.

At the present time some psychoanalysts still believe that most, if not all, diseases are affected by 'psychodynamic factors' and that many skin diseases are primarily caused by the psyche. At the other extreme are those scientific purists who believe that skin diseases are due entirely to biochemical factors, and if a phenomenon cannot be scientifically demonstrated then it probably does not exist. The views of most dermatologists lie somewhere between these extremes."

One danger, for instance, in blaming everything on to ''nerves'' is that insufficient attention is given to other possible disorders, which can even lead to wrong diagnosis and treatment. In his book *More than Skin Deep*, dermatologist Dr Sternberg tells the story of a man who complained of anal itching. With a notable lack of inhibition he seemed constantly to be scratching himself in public.

He went to various doctors and the itching was put down to nervous causes, no doubt some form of sexual repression or frustration. But after several years of enduring this discomfort and at the same time having to feel himself to blame, the man went to a new doctor, who diagnosed pin worms. After treatment for this, the itching disappeared entirely. As he says, this story again illustrates the need for careful examination and the necessity of not accepting a psychological or nervous diagnosis too readily.

There can also be the danger that, having accepted psychological reasons as the cause behind a particular disorder, no other triggers such as allergy or hormone imbalance may be looked for. The flush of rosacea, for instance, was put down in the past to inner feelings of mental and emotional unrest—because of its similarity to blushing.

Now newer findings show that psychological factors probably play very little part, if any, in causing rosacea and that if patients showed signs of embarrassment in their behaviour it was because of the appearance of their faces, and not the embarrassment that caused the appearance. In the same way, the thin-skinned person—physically as well perhaps as emotionally—who tends to blush easily or to suffer from the hot flushes of the menopause is often made far worse when people draw attention to the fact. The flushing in itself causes inner turmoil, not necessarily the other way round.

But perhaps above all it is parents who suffer most from some of the cruder interpretations of Freudian theories which blame certain skin problems in children on mother deprivation, poor parenting, family tension and general emotional neglect.

Says one mother of a child with eczema; ''We were at one time with a specialist who felt that family tensions were the only reason for this condition. When our son first went to the hospital we were asked not to visit him at all, although at his desperate request we of course did. But another child there didn't see his parents for five weeks, and my son's grandmother was asked to leave when he started itching during one of her visits.

"Interviews with this specialist were somewhat like a Nazi interrogation, my husband and I seen separately and placed on chairs in the middle of the room. During one particularly painful session he suggested that we had never wanted the boy as a baby, that we had rejected him, that we did not give him enough love, and that just about everything in our life-style—including moving house and redecorating—was causing his condition.

"Far from being helped, we were reduced to a state of complete panic and despair and from then on, added to the burden of seeing our little boy's suffering, was the extra strain of feeling it was all our fault. This certainly didn't help us cope any better."

Luckily for these parents, when they eventually removed their son from the hospital they learned more balanced views on the subject from another specialist. They realised that though a happy and stable home environment and loving parents are helpful in keeping a skin condition under control, as in any other illness, these are by no means the sole answer.

But there must be other unhappy parents who believe and do not question such accusations against themselves, partly because they think the experts must be right, and partly because the parents of a sick child are particularly prone to guilt and self-accusation. What most of them need is help in getting over these feelings, not more reasons to doubt themselves.

Cause and Effect

Heartening, however, is the growing acceptance of the fact that even when patients (or their close family) present themselves as deeply depressed, anxious, and even highly neurotic, this may be as a very natural *result* of the suffering caused by the skin disorder—a theory hardly considered in those earlier books.

"That patients may feel depressed, resentful or hostile when having to endure recurrent attacks of urticaria for years is not altogether surprising," Dr Whitlock comments.

"Are atopic patients really more hostile and resentful or is this the result of the clinicians subjective interpretation of the patient's mannerisms, behaviour and actual appearance, which to some extent is the direct effect of skin disorder on the facial expression? If, in fact, repressed hostility is an important aspect of the patient's personality make-up, is this the cause or consequence of years of the affliction?''

And talking of acne he says:

"It is not easy to gauge levels of human suffering between one patient and another, but there can be no doubt that severe or even moderate degrees of acne can cause mental disturbance to sensitive adolescents of both sexes.
"There is no reason to believe that their psychological make-up causes the lesions. On the other hand there is more justification for the belief that the lesions can cause anxiety, depression and withdrawal from social life, particularly from contact with the opposite sex.''

For instance Barbara, who is quoted at the beginning of this chapter, feels that she is like two different people with and without her acne. Friends notice the difference, too. As a teenager the spots didn't worry her so much, but when they persisted into her twenties and then returned after she came off the pill at forty, the effect on her personality and life-style was catastrophic.

"I'd gone back to work in an office after having my two children, but I didn't want to go there, I didn't want to go out. I felt everybody was looking at me. I just felt dirty and I felt I either had to cover it up or hide myself away. The spots would just come up over night or in the morning while I was at my desk. My hands broke out in a rash, too, and the acne spread to my chest and the top of my arms.

"I couldn't stand it any more. I tried antibiotics but that didn't help. I got so that I didn't want to cook or do anything and hardly talked to people in case they looked at me. I lost all interest in my appearance, kept eating and got fat. I didn't buy new clothes—what was the point?''

But in the end Barbara hit upon her own salvation. She realised that the acne had cleared both times she was pregnant and when she was on the pill, so she went to her doctor and asked whether she could have a course of oestrogen. Within a fortnight her acne had disappeared, and she will stay on this treatment until after the menopause.

"I felt great, really excited and bubbly," says Barbara. "Other people have noticed a difference and say how much calmer and happier I look. I'm not normally a person who can sit around, but I'd reached the stage when all I wanted to do was hide away. I didn't want to do anything. Now I'm full of energy and wake up every morning looking forward to the day. I even went out without make-up recently. It was so lovely feeling the fresh air on my face."

Another patient, Anne, describes how she had always had eczema on her hands as a child, and how the spectre of her schooldays when no-one would hold hands with her in a ring haunted her for years. But the doctors had always assured her parents that she would grow out of it and in her teens it more or less disappeared.

"Having discovered contact lenses, at seventeen I developed into a very attractive, outgoing young lady. I write now as though this girl is somebody else. I went to university where I got on just as well, being extremely sociable and involved in just about everything which was going on. I had confidence, ability, intelligence, lots of friends and male lapdogs, and thoroughly enjoyed it all.

"Then the eczema reappeared, this time on my face and arms which had never been affected before. All my previous ebullience and confidence evaporated. I was so conscious of my red blotched face I used to carry a small mirror around and peer into it to see how bad it was.

"I refused to wear anything with short sleeves. I stopped wearing make-up, I stopped doing my hair. I found it impossible to talk to people even over the phone. I used to go on my own to lunch, I stopped writing to, phoning and visiting friends. I couldn't bear anybody to touch me. I knew the effect that it was having on everybody, yet I couldn't help it. I became totally absorbed in myself. In the end I had put on two stone in weight, refused to even look in a mirror and ostracised all my friends, my lover and my parents, and stopped going to work.''

Later the eczema subsided again after a stay in hospital. Even though it did not disappear entirely, she adjusted to the problem, became engaged to her boyfriend and returned to her job. But anyone meeting her at the time when her difficulties were at their worst would have thought her highly neurotic and no doubt blamed her skin condition totally on this fact.

As it is, her story illustrates well the delicate balance between cause and effect of emotion and stress and the sort of vicious circle that can build up. Her eczema, she found, was often made worse by various happenings in her life such as an unhappy love affair, university exams, a change in job. But at the same time the very fact that she became itchy, sore and in her eyes unsightly, made her even more depressed and tense.

This vicious circle effect is also shown in the experience of a man with psoriasis. ''There is little doubt that psoriasis in my case was the result of unnecessary anxiety and stress, he says. ''I can clearly remember the devastating effect that psoriasis had on my social life as a young adolescent. I had always been very athletic. I withdrew from sports activities to avoid embarrassment. Adolescents are very sensitive about spots at the best of times. For the young adolescent with psoriasis the effect is devastating.

''The problem moved in a vicious circle of anxiety, frustration and stress to further anxiety, frustration and stress. My parents spared no expense in frantically taking me from one consultant dermatologist to another, and finally to every quack in the countryside, but to no avail. Life became one series of hopes and frustrations.''

On the other hand, another psoriasis patient says: ''I have tried unsuccessfully, even with my specialist's help, to convince my employers that my brain is not affected by the disease. The 'old chestnut' regarding psoriasis being a nervous disease is largely to blame, even though it has been proved beyond doubt that it is genetic and hereditary, and although stress can aggravate it in my case this has proved to be a fallacy."

So there is still a great deal of questioning to be done as to how much effect, if any, stress does have on different skin conditions, and as has already been seen this can be a very difficult thing to assess. In recent times there have been several new studies, but the answers are by no means clear cut.

A controlled study on acne, for instance, at St John's Hospital for Diseases of the Skin in London compared a group of women who had acne with a second group who had other skin disorders affecting the face. From this they found no evidence that the acne was actually caused through pyschological reasons, though they did find that the spots became worse before menstruating and that many of the women were anxious, depressed and suffering from social isolation. The latter they deduced to be a result of the acne, however, and not a cause.

Interestingly, although typically the earlier studies already referred to came to the conclusion that the vast majority of patients with acne showed inhibition and fear of sexuality, in the St John's group of women there was no evidence that either intercourse or marriage improved acne, nor any difference between the two groups interviewed in sexual adjustment after marriage.

Another large study set out to find the significance of psychological symptoms in eczema patients. Reports a psychologist who took part: "My views are that eczema is a particular skin reaction which takes many different clinical forms, and frequently appears in transient episodes and can be provoked or kept going by a number of physical factors such as external irritants, allergies and infections, and is predisposed to in some by genetic factors.

"Inevitably, just as types of eczema vary, so do patients. Their temperaments and ways of dealing with problems and feelings vary as widely as those of any other group of people. But incomplete expression of feelings can contribute to the causation and perpetuation of eczema, particularly feelings of frustration, of resentment and depression.

"It is therefore important we attend to the patient and his feelings as well as his skin. Often psychological stress, involved with a feeling of others not understanding, of feeling isolated, resentful and envious of others not afflicted, anxious about the effect it will have on personal relationships and security of employment, can contribute to a vicious circle."

Two studies on psoriasis patients, one at St Thomas' hospital in London and the other carried out in the patient and parent groups for various skin conditions at the Northampton General Hospital, came to similar conclusions. "Many patients saw psoriasis as a vicious circle," says the report of the first. "For example psoriasis engenders worry or depression which worsens the skin condition, the deterioration leading to further worry."

They also found, as in other studies, that irritation seemed to be worse for the person who felt upset, tense and aggressive towards the condition. Says the dermatologist involved in the group sessions: "Psoriasis is indeed a cause of stress in that we worry about it and worry away at it. In these ways the condition can be a self-stoking fire. If we can find a way of coming to terms with the condition and work out ways of living with it, then we shall dampen the fire, minimise the psoriasis and find life easier and more enjoyable."

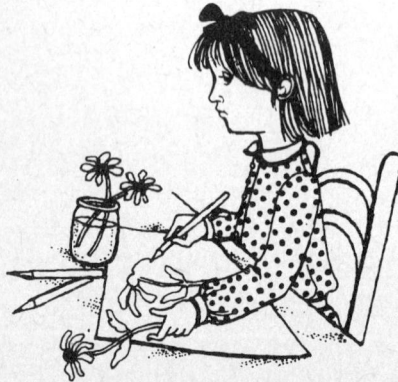

"Don't worry, but keep your child drawing and painting or gardening"

Down with Stress

Whether stress is cause or effect in skin conditions, or if the truth lies somewhere in between, there is no doubt that, as with any illness, to reduce the stress level can only help. On a purely practical plane, the St Thomas' study mentioned above found that if patients felt depressed and hopeless they were less likely to carry out treatments efficiently and consistently.

And as in any other illness, if we are run down or in a low emotional state we are the more vulnerable to ill-health and less able to fight off infection, especially if we are already constitutionally predisposed to a certain ailment. As is mentioned in the next chapter, we are possibly also more liable to become allergic to substances when we are generally 'low'.

How can we deal with the stress that almost inevitably results from a chronic disorder? The dermatologist quoted above found that the group discussions which he held with patients suffering from acne, psoriasis and eczema and their patients, helped many of the people involved. By comparing their own experiences with those of others, by bringing their doubts and fears out into the open and realising they weren't alone, they often felt more relaxed in their approach to their condition and to life in general. Equally helpful was to learn more from the specialist about the physical symptoms and treatment of the disorder.

"The majority of patients who had fought the psoriasis developed a more accepting, peaceful attitude towards it," reports the specialist. "The psoriasis became part of them, and although they still treat the skin they are able to do the treatment with less vehemence and with benefit gained from limited aims and a less hasty approach."

There is a world of difference, of course, between this positive, accepting attitude and the like-it-or-lump it advice: "It's just something you've got to live with" that a few doctors and specialists have been known to give their patients. In fact a doctor's approach towards the patient and the family is all important. A sympathetic attitude which sees nervous aspects as just one possible cause, and as a result of the condition at the same time, is vital.

Many patients are lucky enough to be able to discuss their feelings with their doctor as well as their symptoms. But where this is impossible, it can be invaluable if patients and their families with problems can be referred to interested health visitors, hospital social workers or self-help groups where they can get the support and counselling they need.

The man with psoriasis already mentioned found that later in life he learned to read the physical signs of stress in his own body, and to develop appropriate mental exercises to control. them. Others may find that a new interest such as sailing, painting, music or dance which relaxes and absorbs them, can help minimize their reaction to stresses. For some it may help to join a local class in medication, relaxation or yoga.

Writes one woman with eczema; "One of the greatest sources of relief which I have found is the regular practice of yoga, and in particular, the relaxation techniques. It is little short of miraculous how one can be free of the dread itch for half an hour in 'sarasana' (the corpse position) with the aid of relaxation instructions either on tape or committed to memory. Regular attendance at a yoga class is of enormous help in establishing a routine practice which can be carried out at home with no expense involved."

For those who are close to the person with a skin problem, whether a teacher, a workmate or a member of the family, a relaxed calm approach can also be very helpful. One young woman with eczema says: "I have learnt that it is important to be with someone who does not get over-concerned. Who regards me as being reasonably normal and yet shows kindness when I am feeling sore. Too much serious attention can over-emphasise the problem—and everyone has problems."

Says another adult, looking back on childhood years with eczema: "I think that temperament plays a large part. You cannot alter this, but a calm home gives much benefit, and also to treat this as a natural happening. It's best to encourage people not to talk about the problem in the child's presence. An uncle of mine, when I was about ten, petrified me by discussing what would be done in hospital."

For parents it can be hard not to become tense and anxious

at times when dealing with a sore and itchy child, particularly when that child is still a baby. It won't help these parents to think the disorder is caused by them, but it will help them and the child if they create a happy and secure environment for them all to live in.

One psychiatrist who has worked a great deal with patients and parents in the dermatology department of a large hospital points out in *Exchange* how much of the interaction with a young baby is through skin contact.

"The mother holds the baby securely and rocks it," she says. "She strokes and caresses its skin. She bathes the infant and changes his nappies. She dresses and undresses him. She plays with and moves the infant's limbs. All these interactions through skin contact which both enjoy make the infant feel comfortable; they teach him to experience his own body.

"Then suddenly a condition like eczema appears. Not only will the infant feel uncomfortable but the mother who is normally and naturally anxious at this time of her infants life will be alarmed and distressed, too. At least some of the skin contact on which so much of their interaction depended will have become disappointing and frustrating to both."

It is at this point that tension can start to build up, as the mother feels she is no longer able to make her baby feel content and comfortable and the sore skin begins to act as an emotional wedge between them. However, since the principle treatment of eczema and other skin conditions is the application of soothing medication, this specialist suggests that by gently applying it both mother and infant may get the emotional satisfaction that they would otherwise miss.

To continue to cuddle and show love even if the skin is sore is as important as with any other child, and as she or he grows up interests, friends and an outside life need to be encouraged. Having taken any obvious precautions, parents do not need to overprotect — a normal life is best for the child.

One mother whose son she now describes as a "very large young man of twenty-three" says that she always found the best answer was to distract when he felt uncomfortable or itchy. "Don't worry," she says "but keep your child drawing and painting or gardening or anything so that he forgets to scratch, and keep his mind working on all sorts of subjects so that he forgets himself."

And even if on occasion parents can't help feeling anxiety, the important thing is to try not to show it in front of the child. Says another mother; "If I felt het up, then I'd leave the room. I might go and bang my head against the wall in sheer frustration at times, but I'd do it somewhere else and never in front of my daughter."

A dermatologist recomends good acting as being essential in the family coping with a skin condition. "It is natural to get upset, I quite agree," he says. "But the upset family upsets the patient. Your face is your signal to your child, so try to keep it as calm and cheerful as possible when you are dealing with him. Especially when putting on creams, and so on, avoid gazing anxiously at the skin.

Taking small but positive steps like this will help the patient and the family deal with day-to-day difficulties as they arise without feeling overwhelmed. To be told that it's all due to nerves can leave everyone helpless and at the mercy of causes which seem beyond their reach.

But to see this aspect as just one possible factor in a larger picture, much of which is within our power to control in quite practical ways, can make all the difference to how we cope—and maybe to the condition itself.

5 — What's the Alternative?

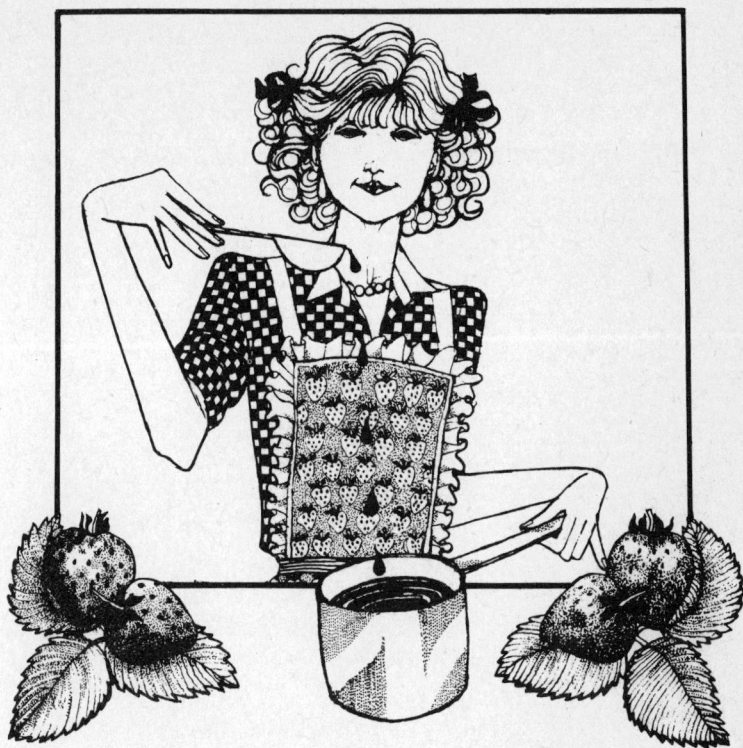

Ancient remedies from strawberry leaves to reindeer antlers have been known to soothe a troubled skin

"Quite by acident we discovered that sea bathing cleared her skin and so this year after our holiday we continued to bath her at home in a strong solution of sea salts which you can buy from health food stores and chemists. Now she is much, much better." *Mother of child with eczema*

"I tried special diets, acupuncture, boracic solutions, lengthy sunshine cruises, antigen injections and hundreds of patent remedies; you name them and I must have tried the lot . . ." *Psoriasis patient*

''Now and again over the past thirty years friends of mine have mentioned their skin complaints. Well, my advice to them is simple—just eat some mustard and cress each day.''

Herbalist

IN recent years there has been an ever-growing interest in alternative medicine, that realm of treatment which lies outside the Western tradition of ''scientific'' medicine and ventures into the more controversial territories of herbs, diet, acupuncture and the like. Having been in the doldrums for quite a time, dismissed by many as somehow cranky or even downright dangerous, fringe medicine is once again being taken much more seriously by people in the West.

Patients with skin conditions are no exception to this trend, and a large number of them and their families are experimenting with various forms of alternative medicine in an effort to put the disorder right. For many the overwhelming attraction of such methods is that they feel they are aiming at the root of the problem—preventing rather than suppressing.

So one mother regularly goes off into the field to collect plantain leaves to turn into soothing preparations for her son's eczema, and another bakes all her own bread, biscuits and cakes with goats' milk. A man goes abroad every year for sun and sea bathing to help his psoriasis, and a teenage girl visits a homoeopath miles from her home to see if he can do anything about her chronic acne.

It follows that such treatments will have wide-ranging effects on a patient's way of life and that of his or her family. Making your own ointments is a lot more difficult than buying them on prescription, and diet can involve complicated and time-consuming procedures checking every label and cooking special dishes. The doctor on the doorstep will also be a lot easier to reach than treatments abroad or even homoeopaths in the next town.

Yet particularly in skin conditions it is understandable that people should want to explore these different and often very ancient methods of treatment. The long-term and so often mysterious nature of many disorders means that patients and their families feel that anything is worth a try, and there is no doubt that in some cases there are very encouraging results.

Even though some people still regard alternative remedies with a great deal of scepticism and perhaps suspicion, there is often a common-sense logic behind them. We are discovering remedies that may once have appeared to be only silly super-stitions are actually based solidly on the medical reality of the body's needs and functions.

For instance, in the light of our reservations about drugs such as steroids and the need to use them sparingly and short-term, it is hardly surprising that many should want to return to the natural preparations made from plants and herbs that have been used traditionally for skin disorders. Though mustard and cress and elder leaves may appear to belong to the class of old wives' remedies, it has to be remembered that many important modern drugs are still derived from plants—the digitalis from foxgloves used in heart conditions, for instance.

Another illustration of changing attitudes is the growing recognition of the important role that diet plays in certain skin conditions, especially eczema. To say that the whole problem is due to "poisons in the blood" put there by faulty food, which then erupts in spots and itches on the skin, is too simplistic; but the fact that allergy and the food we eat can influence certain conditions is beginning to be proved by medical research.

The use of goats' milk is a good example of this. For many years there has been what amounted to an underground army of parents, patients and breeders convinced that eczema and even psoriasis was helped by the use of goats' milk instead of cows'. Surreptitiously they would continue using it in spite of the sceptisism and sometimes downright antagonism of their GP or specialist.

The majority of doctors felt, perhaps understandably, that there was not enough medical evidence to show that any improvement was due to the goats' milk. But the parents, patients and goat owners often saw the evidence with their own eyes.

But now it would seem that what appeared to many as folksy

wishful thinking was in fact based on something more substantial. One leading researcher in the field who has been carrying out studies at a London teaching hospital says: "Twenty years ago cows' milk allergy was regarded as a remarkable rarity. Today the disorder is not only common but the incidence is rising. The number of cases in Britain alone must now run into several thousand, mainly affecting children from the neo-natal period to those in their mid-teens."

Similar studies carried out here and abroad are finding that if "at risk" babies born to parents with eczema are kept off cows' milk and preferably breast fed, they run a far smaller risk of developing the disorder. Taking this even further many doctors are encouraging the mothers to cut cows' milk and allied products out of their diet during pregnancy and during feeding afterwards, and also to wean the child on to a diet excluding cows' milk, substituting soya milk or perhaps goats' milk.

In spite of these findings, opinion is still divided on just how much a change in diet can help other skin conditions. Indeed, advice from different sources can be so conflicting that the patient ends up badly confused.

Acne is a prime example of contradictory ideas. In one book—*Dry Skin and Common Sense* by Dale Alexander—the author recommends that the problems of acne can be put down to improper nutrition. However, read what some of the dermatologists say and you often find a rather different story.

In his book *Dermatology—an illustrated guide* Dr Lionel Fry comments:

"In the past great emphasis has been placed on diet and patients were advised to cut out chocolates, sweets, fatty acids, and to reduce their fat and carbohydrate intake depending on what was fashionable at that particular time. However, there is no real worthwhile evidence as yet to show that manipulation of the diet has a part to play in the management of acne."

Writing in the *British Journal of Medicine* another

dermatologist takes a somewhat cynical approach, advising doctors when treating acne that it is essential to ask patients about their diet, particularly about fats, chocolates and sweets because otherwise they would think the doctor knows very little about acne! He nevertheless feels that there is no convincing proof as to whether diet influences acne one way or another.

Yet still the myth persists, if myth it is, that eating large amounts of chocolate at Easter, or fatty bacon, egg and chips for breakfast, does bring out more spots and pimples, and if the tendency to acne is there that these foods will make it worse.

Perhaps, as so often turns out to be the case, the truth lies somewhere in between the two extremes. Even though for most people a change in diet will not bring about a miraculous recovery, there are some for whom diet and foods like chocolate and chips do make a difference: it may well be worth trying.

It must also be true that the sort of foods under discussion are not the most healthy for anyone, and even less so for a growing adolescent with a tendency to spots. To try to achieve a balanced healthy diet with plenty of fresh green vegetables, salad and fruit can only do good even if it does not magic away the spots completely.

So the most balanced advice would seem to suggest not to become a slave to any diet but, if a particular food does seem to aggravate the acne, to drop it from the diet for a week or so. After a few weeks the food should be reintroduced and effects observed. If acne flares up, then the obvious answer is to avoid that food.

However, many doctors agree that two substances called iodides and bromides contained in certain foods can cause skin eruptions that look very like acne, and can therefore cause skin confusion in diagnosis. Iodides are contained in iodized salt, saltwater fish and shellfish, and both iodides and bromides are in certain drugs such as cough medicines, sedatives and cold medications. It is best, therefore, to avoid excess intake of these while undergoing treatment for acne, although a certain amount is necessary in any healthy diet.

The same uncertainties hang over dietary treatments in psoriasis. Over the years many regimes have been tried and even recommended by doctors, including low-calorie, low-protein, low calcium and fat-free.

There was also the turkey-meat diet, recommended because the inventors were under the impression that this meat contained no tryptophan, a particular amino-acid thought to be a factor in psoriasis. "Interest rapidly diminished, however, when it was discovered that tryptophan was indeed present in turkey" says one specialist writing in *Beyond the Ointment*.

The specialist goes on to say that, though dietary treatment of psoriasis is at a low ebb at this time, the advances made in research into basic chemical changes may soon rekindle it.

"It has been found that there are alterations in psoriatic skin involving a group of fatty acids known as prostaglandins. We do know that prostaglandin level can be changed by strict diets. This has been done in nude mice and hairy rats, which if they are fed too little of the fatty acid building blocks of prostaglandins end up with rapidly growing scaly skin, not altogether unlike psoriasis."

This and other evidence has made more research workers try the effects of giving extra fatty acids, and though no firm conclusions have been reached yet, the research continues. Some doctors also feel that people with psoriasis may be more prone to develop diabetes and raised levels of fats in the blood, and advise that those who have psoriasis should avoid becoming overweight and should cut down on animal fats in the diet.

Diet also comes into the control of other skin conditions. In rosacea, for instance, patients are advised to keep away from alcohol, spicy foods and strong tea and coffee. This is not because, as once thought, that they also suffer from chronic gastritis, but because such foods tend to increase the tendency for the blood vessels in the face to dilate and give a flushed appearance.

Another skin disorder, dermatitis herpetiformis, has been proved beyond doubt to be allied to Coeliac Disease caused by an allergy to gluten in the diet. Remove gluten by using special flours and cereals, and the skin rash disappears.

Urticaria and contact eczema can also be traced on occasion to one particular food or medicine which has been eaten, drunk or simply touched. Shellfish is a common culprit here, but personal reactions can involve foods from tomatoes to eggs to peas to the colouring and flavour additives in food. Skin testing as described in Chapter 2, or elimination diets, can help trace such obvious food allergies, but these are not always reliable and other factors, for instance cold, heat and emotional upset can also play a part.

One dermatologist at Addenbrooke's Hospital in Cambridge describes in *Exchange* how part of this hospital's regular routine when examining patients with eczema, urticaria or contact wealing is to ask for observations on obvious reactions to certain foods, notably swelling of the lips, vomiting or simply consistent refusal.

Any reactions that have been noted are followed by skin tests when a child is old enough to co-operate, although as the specialist explains these must be assessed side by side with careful clinical study since they are not always reliable. As a result of this work, the dermatologist feels that far too many patients restrict their diets unnecessarily, and that a distinction has to be made between allergic reactions to foods in atopic people who happen to have eczema, and a direct effect on the eczema.

Still, this specialist and many others are prepared to consider food allergy as a possible factor in eczema among a small proportion of patients. As has already been touched on at the beginning of this chapter, allergy to cows milk is now clearly established as common in babies and young children.

The researcher involved in the studies mentioned explains:

"At birth the gut is immunologically speaking, highly vulnerable. In infants put to the breast this apparent deficiency is overcome, however. During the first two or three days following birth, the breast secretes not milk but colostrum. Immunologists now believe that babies deprived of colostrum are susceptible not only to bacterial and viral gut infections (and to respiratory infections too) but that their intestine is also more readily penetrated by large molecules of protein in an undiluted form. These pass unimpeded across the unprotected gut and then excite an immune response, as though a foreign protein has been introduced directly into the circulation.''

Like other dermatologists, he would agree that at present there is no reliable laboratory test that will confirm or refute the diagnosis of milk allergy. The only way to confirm suspicions is to exclude cows' milk entirely from the diet for an experimental period, around two weeks. This means in any form, not only as whole milk but as powdered or canned preparations, cheese, butter, cream and yoghurt.

''If the symptoms remit, then milk should be reintroduced into the diet liberally to confirm that an identical set of symptoms is provoked. The case may be considered proven when this manoeuvre has been repeated through three consecutive cycles of withdrawal and challenge.''

The doctor here suggests soya protein as a suitable substitute for the milk, and reassures that the child will come to no harm as long as a reputable and medically recommended brand is used and medical advice is sought over the rest of the diet. Many parents substitute goats' milk in their children's diet, sometimes with remarkable results. Mothers will even make their own cheese, butter and yoghurt and invent special recipes to keep cows' milk out of their children's diet.

Other patients and parents will try the elimination diet described by the doctor to pin down different food offenders. Some adults try the fasting method, whereby they eat nothing and drink only liquid for five days, or live on a mini diet of fruits and vegetables. They then gradually reintroduce foods and watch reactions.

One young woman who started on such an elimination diet after reading Dr Richard Mackarnass's book *Not All In The Mind* found that tea was the culprit with her. After cutting from seven or so cups a day to zero, and also dropping some other foods such as chicken, pork and chocolate, her skin was completely cleared of eczema.

"Two paragraphs in this book gave me the clue," she says. "In the first he explains how most people assume that emotion causes allergy, whereas he believes that the emotion causes only an exhaustion of protective hormones, thus lowering the defences against allergy to a substance that otherwise might not cause any trouble. He then says that you are more likely to react if you have been fighting off a cold or have had an emotional struggle with a loved one, than if you are in robust health, happy and settled." Here, perhaps, is one clue to the link between the emotional and the physical in a skin disorder such as eczema.

Following the work of immunologists and certain dermatologists in the field, dietary treatment of skin disorders now comes under the banner of orthodox treatment of skin disorders as much as that of alternative medicine. But because of the doubts that still exist, many people still go for help outside the medical profession or work on their own hunches.

One couple took their two small children with eczema to a herbalist who, besides providing herbal ointment and infusions to drink, also recommended a vegan diet which cut out all animal products, including eggs and cheese. The children live on ground brown rice, pulses, seeds, nuts, honey and vegetables—and their skins are completely clear.

Eating Naturally

In fact many of the alternative methods of treatment, including herbalism, homoeopathy and naturopathy, place changes in diet high on their list of priorities. This does not necessarily mean that the person is allergic to any particular food, but that the body and the skin in particular benefit from a healthy diet that excludes man-made additives and includes natural foods such as brown whole-meal flour, honey, brown sugar, plenty of vitamins and fresh fruit and vegetables.

Once you start delving, it is surprising how many of today's treatments were used in rather more primitive form hundreds and even thousands of years ago. In his book *Living with Your*

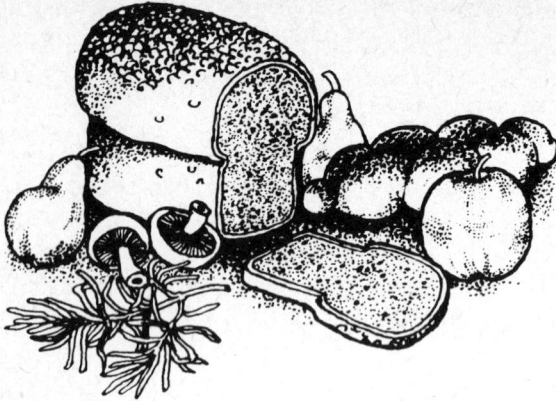

The whole body, and the skin in particular, will benefit from a healthy diet

Psoriasis, George Sava relates an old legend about an Indian Princess whose brown skin became covered in white patches. Physicians and herbalists from far and wide went to work, but none could find a cure until a wandering sage came to the palace.

He ground some black seeds and mixed the resulting powder with wild bee's honey and said that after rubbing the ointment into the paler patches of her skin, the princess should lie in the sun. Within a month she was cured. As the author points out, this happened fourteen centuries BC in India. Now it is known that the princess's disease was vitiligo. And the treatment of honey mixed with *Ammi majus* seeds powder—the present day *psoralens*—followed by exposure to the sun, is more or less the exact description of modern photochemotherapy, the only difference being that now we use crystalline extracts from the plants, and ultraviolet radiation instead of the sun's rays. In his book this author also describes more obscure and yet apparently equally successful ancient Oriental folk cures, such as teas and pastes made from the antlers of reindeer—which interestingly enough are formed with the same keratin which goes into the horny layer of the human skin. He describes the case of one girl who for three months drank tea made of thin slices of antler whenever she felt thirsty, and covered her patches of psoriasis with a paste made from honey, dry seeds, leaves of Bishop's weed and antler powder every night before going to bed. By the end of the third month practically all her psoriasis was clear.

Nearer to home, one eczema sufferer recommends strawberry leaves, another comfrey, and a psoriasis patient personally vouches for the use of old-fashioned dock leaves. "It is well known in rural areas that if one is stung by nettles, rubbing with a dock leaf will instantly reduce pain and swelling," he says. "I have used this on occasions and it works every time. I have also been told that there are references in some of the mediaeval alchemy books to concoctions of dock leaves for curing skin abnormalities."

In his book *A Guide to Alternative Medicine*, which covers sixty different therapies, Donald Law mentions *urtica dioica* which the Romans in particular used against chills, feverish colds, bleeding, bladder troubles, skin diseases and as a spring tonic.

"It has been shown to contain silica, calcium, chlorophyll, Vitamins A and C, iron, a substance similar to histamine, formic acid and a glucose similar to quinine. It is the common stinging nettle!"

Today millions of people have turned to herbal medicine in preference to all other forms of healing, he says. In most countries there is an association from which you can get information about herbalism and those who practice it, and in the shops there are dozens of creams and ointments containing various herbal extracts. But as Donald Law points out, if you decide to become your own herbalist great care should be taken.

"Clearly no-one should pick out a herb and use it without reading up its functions, how it was used by herbalists historically, how much and how often, etc."

Naturopathy also includes the use of herbalism and dietary reform, very often in conjunction with baths and sun treatment. All over Europe, spas with their mineral rich waters have long been known to help in certain skin disorders, and a change in climate can also be useful.

So seriously is this type of treatment taken abroad in countries such as Norway, Sweden, Denmark and Finland, that the health ministries have their own travel agencies and doctors will prescribe "health tours". The main centres for skin disorders are in Israel, Yugoslavia and Bulgaria, where people can enjoy a holiday while receiving their treatment, staying in a cross between a hotel and a hospital with trained medical staff on hand.

Though the most dramatic results have been seen in patients suffering from psoriasis, these centres also claim to be able to help patients with other skin disorders. A main area for climato therapy, as it is called, is around the Dead Sea in Israel. The climate is dry and mild and because the Dead Sea area is well below sea level the sunlight reaching it is low in ultra-violet rays.

Just as important, the waters of the Sea itself contain ten times more chemicals than ordinary sea waters, and some of these chemicals such as magnesium are said to be very beneficial to the skin. In the same way Bulgaria has a good climate, and its waters are rich in chemicals such as iodine and magnesium. Both countries also have natural springs and spas to which people with varying ailments flock. In Yugoslavia there are three centres run by the government especially for skin disorders. You can find out more about these from the various tourist offices.

Sun on its own is known to have a beneficial effect on a few conditions including psoriasis, acne and eczema—although, as we've already seen, for some it can make a condition worse, particularly in those who are light sensitive. As with so many therapies, it is a matter of careful trial and error.

But in psoriasis the effects are almost always good. Two patients describe their improvement after a visit to Spain. "I found this quiet beach where I could get into my swimming costume without thinking people were staring at me. I suppose it was the sun, the air and the fact I was relaxed, but I could see the psoriasis fading away," says one.

"I spent a total of six weeks at Calpe near Benidorm and spent most of my time on the beach," says another patient. "At the end of six weeks I found I was completely clear of psoriasis on my body. I felt that the sun, olive oil and constant sea bathing in this part of the Mediterannean with its high salt content, all contributed."

Acupuncture is another branch of alternative medicine through which many patients have found help, often combined with other treatments such as oesteopathy. One mother describes the change it has worked on her son's eczema after years of suffering from the complaint:

"Although he has not had the needles, the oesteopathy he has received through the twelve pressure points of this Chinese system have given him a new energy and he is becoming completely revitalised," she says. "We hardly know him for the boy he has been for so long now—is it five years, even six?"

The theory behind acupuncture is that there are meridian lines passing through the body which carry a life force and are distinct from the actual physical nervous system. This force must function without any hindrance for bodily health to be maintained.

Treatment can be by needle, finger pressure, moxa heat or electric stimulus to one or more of the acupuncture points on the surface of the body. Diagnosis is traditionally by four methods: looking, listening, asking questions and palpating. Deviations from the normal are sought in skin colour and texture, heat, cold, moisture.

"Carefully investigated are the Chinese pulses: on each wrist the acupuncturist can feel and determine the vitality of six different organs and functions of the living body," says one patient. "Pulse information is used both to help analyse the patient and to monitor progress after treatment is given.

"Prevention of illness is the keynote: living in harmony with the laws of nature as expressed in the philosophy of integration and wholeness, respect for change and knowledge of the self. Given ill health, the patient and not the disease will be analysed, cause determined and treatable imbalances evaluated."

In this sense there is some overlap between acupuncture and homoeopathy, a system which has on the whole crossed the barrier between alternative and orthodox medicine and which is practiced by many conventionally trained general practitioners.

One psoriasis patient who has experimented with homoeopathy says that at its base is the philosophy that patients are treated as individuals and their whole personality must be taken into account when prescribing medication. Each person has within him a vital force to survive and this force is encouraged by homoeopathic medicines and not dampened down as by modern drugs.

"The minimal dose is the secret of homoeopathic prescribing, and not as much medicine as possible to drown the disease," he explains. "It is therefore understandable that homoeopathy has its best results with children whose systems are not clogged up with a variety of medicaments."

An eczema patient, who had been on steroid treatment for sixteen years before starting homoeopathic treatment, found nevertheless that she was greatly helped. "The homoeopathic small doses (called potencies) of natural remedies are used to stimulate the body's own defensive and curative processes," she says.

"Homocopathy is based on the principle that like should be treated with like and that sickness is not a localised thing but involves the whole person. The treatment consists of lovely cooling lotions as well as various pills and powders. I saw the doctor often and regularly as he experimented to find out what suited me best."

The remedies used can be animal, vegetable and mineral. Homoeopaths do use herbs and botanical medicines but usually only after potentisation. They also use drugs such as morhphine, cocaine and even arsenic, but again in their potentised form and therefore no longer poisonous. Again, there is an association where those interested can obtain information—the address is given at the end of this book.

Hypnosis is another branch of fringe treatment which in many instances is being taken under the umbrella of orthodox medicine, and there is at least one dermatologist who works with hypnotism and sees its beneficial effects when applied to various skin conditions.

In his book *Psychophysiological Aspects of Skin Disease* Professor F. A. Whitlock mentions particular cases where hypnosis relieved patients of their itching sensation. One possibility, he says, is that in the relaxed, anxiety-free state of hypnosis either itch thresholds can be raised, or receptivity and response be inhibited. It is also known that hypnosis can change body temperature, which in turn could affect the state of the skin. Thirdly, he says, one has to consider the possibility that hypnosis might affect a centrally caused itching state, although hard evidence for this is lacking at present.

He also records how hypnosis has helped people with various allergic conditions and even, surprisingly, icthyosis. One man improved in warm weather and was worse in winter. Under hypnosis the patient was given suggestions that his skin was warm and comfortable and after a month or so he improved, despite cold weather.

Warts are another example of a trying skin condition which can apparently be improved or even cured under hypnosis. But as with all cases, success does appear to depend very much on the patient being a good subject for hypnosis, and on the depth of the trance. Like any skin condition, warts are also known to clear up quite spontaneously, and it would be difficult to prove conclusively whether the hypnosis actually charmed the disappearing warts away or whether this was simply co-incidence.

Remedies for All

There are many more branches of alternative medicine and fringe treatments which patients have reported as being helpful. In his book Donald Law includes several obscure ones such as colour therapy, when lights are shone through special coloured filters on to the body (blue is apparently best for skin troubles), and "winding" in which the patient is wrapped up in damp towels with oak bark, and is then fed honey sweetened herbal teas!

A whole chapter is devoted to biochemistry, and the use of tissue salts. One man whose wife has psoriasis writes: "She had it to a chronic degree on both hands and had needed to wear cotton gloves for more than seven years because there was no whole flesh on her hands. I bought a copy of a book about biochemistry and studied it, and as a result my wife used a dosage of tissue salts.

"What happened was truly amazing. Seven days after commencing treatment there were no new outbreaks, and with the passing of a further seven days the skin was almost whole: the scars were barely visible. That treatment ceased after approximately one month and for a further two weeks nothing happened. But then a small outbreak appeared on the palm of the left hand so a lesser dosage than the original was started and the trouble is held in check."

The author of *Dry Skin and Common Sense* is convinced that cod liver oil is the answer to all skin problems, as to most other illnesses, including arthritis. He suggests that if cod liver oil becomes a part of daily living then most conditions including acne, eczema and psoriasis, will go away.

His theory that the cod liver oil, apart from supplying various health-giving nutrients such as vitamins, minerals and fatty acids, also lubricates the body from within sounds plausible enough. So though the claim that it will cure everything under the sun appears somewhat sweeping, there can be no harm in giving it, too, a try.

Cures recommended by patients themselves are legion. One person swears by Brewers' Yeast, another by a teaspoonful of sunflower oil night and morning. One mother rubs capsules of Vitamin E into her child's skin every day and another found that the minerals in a certain stream in Scotland did the trick. One woman improved after X-ray treatment, one baby on a diet of mashed potatoes.

"The turning point came for us when Andrew was eight months old and we went for a day to the sea," writes a mother. "I had been told by an old woman about the value of seaweed to the skin and rubbed his legs with this very smelly seaweed. Within two days the scales had gone!"

The list is endless—and here is where one of the dangers of such treatments can lie. If one isn't careful it is possible to get caught up on a never-ending treadmill of experiment, trying first this method, then that diet, then this remedy with hope followed by desperate disappointment if the promised success isn't achieved.

As the psoriasis patient quoted at the beginning of this chapter adds: "I must have tried the lot, but always in partial ignorance of their effects and whether I might in reality be harming myself. Most were of benefit in the short term for periods of a few months, and initially I had an occasional total disappearance of the scales, but with each major return of my psoriasis came a shattering despondency, a realisation of failure and futility. Luckily another straw almost always drifted by when all seemed lost."

"In the early days we grasped at any straw that might provide a cure," says the husband of a woman with psoriasis. "The mind shut to reality will not accept the possibility of a life-long relationship with psoriasis. That realisation came well after the first frantic attempts to rid ourselves of the scourge. Like most at the beginning, we sought out every medical aid to rid ourselves of the condition.

"Then there were the creams and ointments, some recommended by friends, some proprietary brands and others herbal with a touch of the witch doctor about them. Oh yes, and then we asked, everywhere we went we asked. We spent a year and a half behind the Iron Curtain; we asked there. They were very keen to help and we tried their treatment, but to no avail. We spent four years in Germany and sampled their 'cure' too—even three weeks in hospital—and recently, of course, the Dead Sea cure. I don't think we will ever stop trying, but there came a time when we stopped deluding ourselves."

As this couple eventually found, the answer lies in the general attitude with which one approaches new treatments, alternative or otherwise. If the patient and the family can develop a philosophical frame of mind, which hopes for the best but isn't too cast down when it doesn't come, then to keep trying can be helpful to everyone.

After all, you may not always be looking for a complete cure but for some improvement, and experiences show that very often this does happen. If hopes aren't set too high, then the lift and sense of optimism that patient and family can feel from trying a new treatment may in themselves be good for the disorder.

"Even if in the end it doesn't make much difference, it can be really rewarding to know you are doing something to help yourselves rather than just sitting back and letting it happen," says one mother of a boy with eczema.

One mother who herself had eczema and now has two children with the disorder, however, remembers her childhood as one dreary succession of dietary and other regimes. Her mother, a health food expert and cook, was meticulous in seeing that the diets were kept to correctly, yet they made little difference to the eczema.

"What they did affect was my personality," she says. "I remember becoming increasingly withdrawn and unhappy, and have really only got over the psychological effects in recent years. In consequence I try to keep my own children's lives as normal as possible.

"It's the sweeping statements of some enthusiasts that turns me away. The suggestion that just because a certain type of treatment helps one person it will help everyone I know from experience just isn't true."

A diet that shows definite results will be worth pursuing. But if it doesn't make much difference then the added strain placed on a child by banning favourite foods will be unfair, simply making a rather difficult life even more difficult for no good reason.

There can be other dangers. In recent years doctors have been discovering cases of rickets among babies put on special diets without proper guidance from a nutritional expert or doctor. It is also important to buy goats' milk from a reputable goat breeder.

Another complication is that the fluctuating nature of most skin ailments can make it very hard to judge whether a particular treatment is helpful or not. It is always just possible that a rash was going to clear anyway in a natural remission. And as one specialist points out, though the herbalist or goat breeder will advertise his or her successes, the failures get overlooked.

So the parent and the patient start blaming themselves if the latest treatment does not work, and new tensions and problems can be added to the already existing ones. If you are not careful, the whole of life can become a never-ending battle to find the elusive treatment that will bring about a cure.

"We have tried numbers of different treatments including herbal creams and tablets, a goats' milk diet, a vegetarian diet followed by a vegan diet, and even a wheat-free diet when all the bread I baked came out looking like Yorkshire batter!" says one mother whose attitude remains realistic.

"But even though none of these did much good in the long run, we don't regret the effort. Having tried a treatment, even if it doesn't work, gives you more peace of mind and acceptance. At least we haven't got that nagging feeling in the back of our minds that maybe if we did this or did that, then our son would get better."

It also means a few less mysteries to be added to the mysteries that are already there.

6 — The Child and the Family

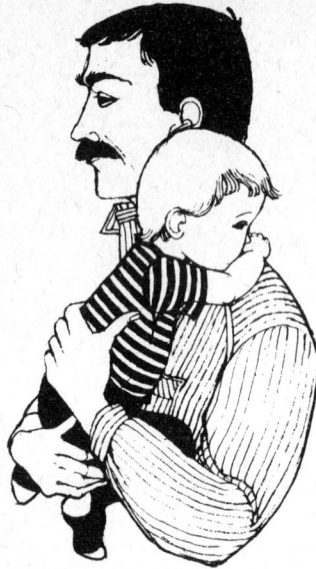

The child whose skin is sore will want to be cuddled as much, if not more, than any other

"My pretty daughter, who had previously had such a healthy skin, looked a mess . . . I think I found the psoriasis more difficult to accept than Kathy did, although I knew she might get it. At first when I saw her body covered in spots I felt like crying."

A mother

"Children's reactions—often through innocence—could be the most hurtful. I lost count of the times I was asked 'what's wrong with your hands?' "

Adult looking back

"Having eczema is not very nice because you keep on scratching and it hurts, and your clothes stick to you. And sometimes my legs are so dry I just can't straighten them."

Tessa, aged seven

ONE of the most comforting facts for parents to hang on to when their child suffers from a long-term skin condition is that there is every hope it will improve, if not completely clear, as he or she grows older and the body and skin mature.

This is particularly true of atopic eczema. In one study following the progress of children treated in a hospital out-patient's department, eighty-two percent were clear by the age of fifteen. In another study on children who were treated by their family doctor, ninety-six percent were clear by twelve. In a large proportion of cases the eczema lasts only through babyhood, which is why it is often described as "infantile" eczema.

It is for this reason as much as any other that children with a skin disorder need to be encouraged to lead as active and as normal a life as possible, because when the skin is healthy again it is so important that the mind and personality should be, too. So however tempting it may be to coddle and over-protect, instead the children should be helped within certain limitations to do the same things as any others.

Often, in fact, they will need little encouragement. Both parents and dermatologists have noticed how generally bright, friendly and outgoing many such children are—a result perhaps of the extra amount of love and care that they may of necessity have received. They also often seem to have a natural energy, which can even make them "hyperactive" as babies but as they grow older this can be channelled into any number of activities and enthusiasms. Perhaps, too, the very fact that they have had problems to deal with from a very early age gives them a gritty sort of courage and determination which means they will tackle almost anything given half a chance.

The experience of many parents bears this out. Writes one mother: "My son is now a very large young man of twenty-three, a teacher who specialises in physical education. But he suffered terribly from eczema as a child. We survived it, and so did he. He is emotionally very stable with a lively sense of humour and far more friends than most people."

Says another: "Cathy is now in her first year at university and coping well with life. It makes me realise just how great an improvement there has been, from a child struggling painfully to school with stiff, bent knees, to Cathy as she is today.''

Mention chronic skin disorders in babies and young children, and most people will think of eczema. But psoriasis, although it is generally thought of as an adult disorder, affects around one thousand and seventy-five thousand children below the age of ten in this country, and approximately one third of patients develop the condition between the ages of ten and nineteen—a proportion even as babies.

There are also the rare, but often serious skin conditions like *epidermolysis bullosa*. Blisters form spontaneously on the baby's skin from birth, and later can result from any pressure on the skin, even a loving cuddle or hug.

Some skin abnormalities are more common in infants than in adults. Children are very prone to have warts, for instance, and fungal infections of the scalp, body and feet. Cold sores and impetigo may frequently erupt; babies will be found with various rashes round the nappy region and the face; and there can be a tendency towards urticaria or hives which persists throughout childhood.

There are various reasons for these differences. Though many think of a baby as just a small version of an adult, he or she may have different problems medically and this is especially true of the skin. When first born the child will have been strongly influenced by the mother's hormones and chemicals, and in some cases may have excessive hair, small red spots or even occasionally acne, though most of these problems are naturally resolved once the hormone imbalance settles down.

On top of this the skin has not developed into its mature state and does not have the same protection against bacteria and other outside agents—for instance wind and sun—as that of the older child or adult. Because of the immature state of the baby's or young child's immune system, which protects against allergy and infection, he or she is more likely to be susceptible to the virus infections of the wart or cold sore, or fungal infections such as athlete's foot which causes the skin on the toes to become sore and itchy.

Some of the reasons for this vulnerability in skin disorders in early childhood are to do with the life pattern at this age. Before being toilet trained a young baby's skin is likely to become wet and soiled if nappies are not changed frequently enough, and various rashes can develop. Though more frequent changing of nappies and cleansing, plus baby lotions and creams such as zinc ointment, may clear these up, diagnosis by a doctor can also be helpful.

Nappy rash can be due to ammonia in the urine or an infection from the yeast Candida, which also causes the white plaques of thrush in a baby's mouth. The sensitive skin may be reacting to irritants in soap or talc, or to detergent left in nappies which have not been rinsed thoroughly enough. At times just the process of crawling can irritate the skin on hands and knees, and the baby and toddler will be particularly at the mercy of dirt and dust to be found at ground level.

As children grow up, their vulnerability to some extent remains connected with the sort of life they lead. At play and at school they mix closely with so many children that they are almost destined at some time or another to pick up infections such as the sores called impetigo, the ingrowing wart on the foot called verruca or the normal run of childhood illnesses from measles to chickenpox. Ringworm is another fungal infection, and further hazards are the infestations of scabies in the skin, or lice and nits in scalp and hair.

Nasty though these skin problems may sound and can often be, they are no longer the scourge they once were. There are simple and successful treatments for them all, and whereas something like lice and nits could once take months to control and cause great social distress to a whole family, modern lotions, and help from school health teams, make this particular difficulty far less traumatic.

But of course there are still some skin conditions in infancy which are not short-term or easy to control, and which can cause prolonged problems for the child and the parents. The most common of these are psoriasis and eczema. Both are hereditary disorders and though it is possible for a child to be the first in the line, you can usually trace some relative who has suffered from either condition or, in the case of eczema, from the closely allied asthma, hayfever or rhinitis.

A complicating factor in estimating the number of young sufferers from psoriasis is that it is frequently misdiagnosed and initially called eczema, athlete's foot or even chickenpox. As a dermatologist explains in the Psoriasis Association magazine *Beyond the Ointment*, a rash which appears on the nappy region and even looks like psoriasis may turn out to have been provoked by a thrush infection and to have no other significance. But in the infant of a family where someone is a psoriasis patient the rash may prove to have been true psoriasis, the child later developing the typical scaly patches.

"Psoriasis of the usual type rarely begins before the age of four or five," she says. "The onset is often an outbreak of what is called *guttate* psoriasis, *gutta* being the Latin word for drop. Guttate is an accurate description of the rash, which consists of many very small scaly patches affecting the trunk and limbs and sometimes the scalp. Sometimes there a few rather larger patches, or such patches in time develop.

"This type of rash often follows an infection, often one caused by streptococci in the throat; usually the rash clears well, but in some children patches will linger indefinitely. It is somewhat commoner in girls than in boys and may or may not itch. If a child has a tendency to tonsilitis the rash may come back with each attack and it is in these cases that the removal of the tonsils may be advised. Fortunately, however, serious psoriasis and the linked form of arthritis, are exceedingly rare."

Eczema in the child is most commonly of the atopic type already described, and can vary from small sore patches behind the ears or knees, to a weeping rash which covers the whole body. In other babies and young children the eczema is of the seborrhoeic type, which may start with a crusty "cradle cap" on the scalp, the scaly rash later affecting the eyebrows, cheeks and ears and sometimes extending to the chest, neck and even nappy area. This usually clears up quite quickly, however, with correct treatment.

Urticaria or contact wealing in infants, caused by allergy or sensitivity to some substance or food either touched or eaten, can also be confused with eczema, but it will usually disappear once the culprit has been found. In a really serious case the allergy will take the form of oedema, when there is not only inflammation of the skin but also swelling of lips and eyelids and sometimes tongue and throat. The latter can be dangerous as it can cause suffocation, and prompt medical treatment is necessary.

The general treatment of psoriasis and eczema for children is similar to that for adults, but on the whole the creams should be used rather more sparingly, and some are not suitable for children's sensitive skins at all. In psoriasis, for instance, dithranol should be used with special care, and if steroid ointments are applied at all only the weaker hydrocortisone is suitable, particularly on the face and more sensitive areas such as the groin. The more dramatic treatments such as methotrexate and PUVA are not generally recommended for children.

In eczema the same sort of rules apply, with stronger steroids being avoided as much as possible and never used on the face or sensitive areas of the body. Bandages impregnated with tar or zinc can be particularly useful because they also protect from scratching, and daily baths with emulsifying ointment or oilatum instead of soap help lubricate and moisturise the skin.

Anti-histamine syrups or tablets help to ease the irritation of eczema, urticaria and psoriasis. Their sedative effects give the children (as well as their long-suffering parents!) much needed rest at night, and though this can lead to some drowsiness in the day, on the whole the benefits outweigh the drawbacks and there are no other worrying side effects.

Cotton clothing and bedding is found to be best for most children with a skin disorder, partly because it is naturally softer and less irritating than nylon or wool, and also because it allows better ventilation to the skin. For babies an all-in-one suit with mittens attached can be helpful in protecting the skin from scratching.

Many parents try the various "alternative" methods of

treatment mentioned in the previous chapter, often finding particular success with homoeopathy and special diets. The danger can be that the child's life becomes too dominated by such experiments, until a whole family's existence revolves round them.

This can be especially true with diet and with allergy avoidance in general, so parents need to balance the general inconvenience and hardship for the children in banning, for instance, much loved foods or pets, against the good effects this has on the skin condition. Particularly with young babies, specialists stress that they need a balanced and nutritious diet and any changes need checking with doctor or dietician.

However, evidence from patients and their families—and more recently from the medical profession—shows that diet can play an important role in a condition like eczema. As was mentioned in the previous chapter, new research has shown that when a baby is obviously at risk of developing eczema because one or both parents have it, breast feeding may build up certain defences. It may also help if the feeding mother keeps off cows' milk and products herself, and maintains a similar diet during pregnancy.

At the Institute of Child Health in London experiments have gone even further, by keeping these "at risk" children away from obvious allergy-provokers such as feathers in pillows or eiderdowns, house dust, pollen from flowers and wool in bedding or clothing. This was kept up well into the first year. The babies were carefully weaned on to a non-cows' milk solid diet using a recognised soya milk as substitute. Other well known allergy causers such as eggs and wheat were also excluded from the diet.

Using as controls other "at risk" babies who received no such avoidance regime, the first set of babies showed a marked decrease in the development of eczema. Nothing has been proved conclusively as yet, and there are some who regard such findings with a degree of scepticism. But for parents with eczema already in the family it is encouraging to know that there are measures which can be taken and which might help.

The way in which psoriasis is passed on through families is

still not clear. As a specialist explains: "Largely because we have no good method of picking out those people who have the tendency to it before they actually develop signs of it, and since the onset may be late in life and the actual rash minimal, many people will have died without being noted as suffering from psoriasis.

"In general, however, there is no doubt that having one parent with psoriasis will increase the chances of a child's developing the condition, and that having two such will increase them further. It is also probable that with such a background the psoriasis will tend to arise fairly early in life."

The actual hereditary mechanism in eczema is not fully understood either. It may be that parents pass on some defect in the child's immunological system, which means that he or she has a greater tendency to develop allergies to many substances. In asthma this will lead to wheezing and coughing; in hayfever to running eyes and nose; and in ezcema to an itchy, inflamed skin.

As with any hereditary condition, parents with a skin disorder may hesitate about having children at all when they consider the difficulties it has caused them, and perhaps still does. In forms of *epidermolysis bullosa* one child born with the condition will almost certainly be followed by other children with it. But since in skin conditions such as psoriasis, eczema and acne it is never certain that this will be passed on, doctors do not recommend that a couple need deny themselves children.

Another aspect to bear in mind when considering any risk is that experience of a condition may actually help parents deal better with the day-to-day problems that can arise. The child, too, may be able to understand and cope better.

Says one mother whose daughter developed psoriasis when she was five: "We were fortunate in that Katy was able to accept the psoriasis fairly easily. My niece, who lives nearby, already had psoriasis and to Katy it was just another illness, like measles or chickenpox."

Says an adult eczema patient: "My husband who has seen me at my worst with eczema would not consider it a reason for depriving ourselves of a family. In fact I think that parents who have eczema themselves are likely to be far more capable of coping with their children's eczema than those who have not experienced it themselves.''

Feelings of Guilt

There is no doubt however that, particularly if their child's skin conditions does come as a complete surprise and is not something they have consciously prepared for, many parents suffer feelings of extreme guilt and inadequacy at what they see their children going through.

Again, this may be the case with all illnesses in children. But there is something about skin disorders which, quite apart from the hereditary aspects, seems to reflect badly on the family, perhaps mainly because of the associations already described with poor parenting, neglect, dirt and infection.

Says a psychiatrist experienced in dermatology among children: ''When one comes to think of it in detail, one realises that it would be very surprising indeed if parents of these children did not sometimes experience such emotions.

''To start with, the feelings of inadequacy. Firstly, the cause of conditions like eczema and psoriasis is not known exactly, nor is the reason why they become chronic in some patients. Secondly, there is no known treatment which can confidently be expected to clear the eczema in all patients equally well and equally quickly.

''Therefore if treatment which clears the condition satisfactorily in one child does not achieve the same good result in their own child, parents may be left wondering whether the lack of success is their fault. In other words, are they inadequate?''

The psychiatrist goes on to explain that it is only a short step from there to feeling guilty towards the child, and unless parents keep calm and continue to show that they love their child a very vicious circle of feelings may build up. Attempts to find successful treatments may become too determined, the child may be told too often and too desperately not to scratch or to go out to play or occupy himself better indoors, and in due course feelings of inadequacy and guilt may increase.

"They may be over still not finding a remedy, or for disturbing the child's routine and normal growing up processes. They may stem from seeming to tell the child off and making demands on him, when in fact the parents' actions were prompted by concern, pity and sympathy for the child's suffering.

"Perhaps the most important single point for coping successfully with these feelings is for parents not to take them at face value, thinking they really are inadequate or have done something they should not have done or omitted to do something they should have done.

"Instead they must always keep it firmly and absolutely clearly in their minds that these feelings are aroused by the child's condition and to make sure that the child understands this and knows it, too."

Inevitably also, the parent is likely to be upset by the sight of the child's sore and damaged skin, and then feel guilty about this. It is only natural to want people to admire one's child and on occasion to see him or her as an extension of ourselves. When people gape in amazement, remove their own children from contact or turn away in embarrassed silence, it is bound to hurt.

Says a dermatologist: "Of course, all the pram comment and enthusiastic advice that one receives adds so much to the strain of coping with the patient. All parents love to push their child out for other people to coo over. But when nobody coos and all we receive is a lot of advice about what one should do and what one should not do, we feel terribly bereft.

"One is feeding the baby wrongly ('don't give him lemon juice,' 'do give him lemon juice,' 'try goats' milk') one is doing this wrongly and that wrongly. People are only too willing to provide their advice from their experience and imagination, perhaps allaying their own anxiety by doing so."

The end result of all these pressures can be that the child himself becomes confused about who or what his parents' distress is directed against. He may come to feel he is an inadequate or even unacceptable person because he does not respond to everybody's efforts. In the end he may come to feel that he can be of no good to anyone until he is free of his skin condition.

Looking back on his eczema as a child, one adult patient says: "I think it's important not to agonise over whose 'fault' it is. I went through periods of thinking I had it because I was bad, or because my parents were perpetuating it. My parents felt by turns that I must be able to stop it if I wanted to, or that they must in some conscious way be encouraging it.

"It may simply be that the physical side of a condition like eczema has to be acknowledged, and that it doesn't help to think that that tiny bit of extra effort or psychological insight on your part will cure it."

One-time child patients remembering their feelings like this can offer great insight to present-day parents as to how a son or daughter with a skin disorder feels. It is often difficult for very young children to rationalise their problems when they are face to face with them, but later they can see and explain them more fully.

Remembers one psoriasis patient: "In the years between eight and thirteen psoriasis spread to all parts of my body, mercifully the covered parts, with patches on all my limbs. It was a shock when at age eleven we had to wear only shorts and plimsoles for physical training.

"All eyes seemed to be upon me, and all sorts of teasing took place. I must, however, say something in defence of my classmates—I doubt whether any of them had seen or heard of psoriasis before.

"Most psoriatics will be able to report similar situations, but the point I would make is that children suffer much more than adults because they do not have control over the factors which cause so much anguish. I often ponder how much worse it would have been for a girl with less covering clothes."

Recalls a woman who was just such a little girl: "Throughout my childhood I tried to conceal my skin when it became unsightly. I remember in primary school wearing woollen cardigans over short-sleeved summer dresses—just to cover my raw arms. Of course, the cardigans created more irritation, but that was better than the shame of others seeing the state of my skin. Little girls, even at the age of nine or ten, are very sensitive as regards appearance."

Another patient remembers how much ordinary things like soap, water, salt, washing-up liquid and juice in orange peel hurt her sore hands. She appeals to all adults on behalf of those who are children now not to under-estimate the level of real suffering involved.

"Be patient with grubby hands, missed piano practices and woollen sock grumbles," she asks. "And do not take school reports at face value. Children can be so cruel to one another and a child's life at school may not be easy. Physical rejection is a hard thing to live with, and work is the first thing to suffer if the child is putting up with endless taunts of 'Ugh, aren't your hands horrid? You can't play with us'."

An education welfare officer who has made a study of the effects of cosmetic handicap in the child at school, stresses the importance of parents' positive attitudes towards a child's disability in the early years of growing up.

"What adjustments a visually different child makes in the first instance is the product of family reaction," he stresses. "If the family accept and love the child, including the differences he may possess, then he will likely develop in a natural, supportive environment, to become a well adjusted individual.

"Within the family it is crucial that the pre-school child has developed the necessary emotional attachments to parents (or adult figures), and of marginally less importance to brothers and sisters. The child's later relationships with people will very much depend upon the experiences of these first few years."

This holds good for any child, but for the child with some form of blemished skin there are particular steps to take which can help. However sore the child, he or she needs to be cuddled and caressed quite as much, if not more than, any other. Though he may not look beautiful to some outsiders, he needs the reassurance of admiring looks and compliments as he grows up.

Says one mother: "I found that when Matthew was small it was helpful and kind to kiss his poor raw patches the same way that one would comfort any small child that had fallen down and cut a knee. I think this was important because it didn't make him feel there was anything untouchable about his skin.''

Since so many skin conditions irritate, particularly eczema and urticaria but also on occasion psoriasis, the young child's scratching will raise many problems. Although it was once the rule to go so far as to tie a young child's hands in splints or against the side of the cot at night to stop scratching, attitudes have changed in recent years.

Says one dermatologist who recommends free scratching. ''It is natural for them to itch and therefore it is equally natural for them to resolve this. Hence, if one develops an atmosphere in which as much as possible the scratching is understood and at times even encouraged, the child himself feels accepted and more secure—and in fact has been proved to scratch less, particularly at night. Also, of course, guilt feelings about scratching later on in life are lost, too.''

It is often very hard for parents and adults involved with the child to condone scratching. Explains a mother: ''The specialist said that our attitude would make a lot of difference. It meant stopping oneself a dozen times a day from saying: 'Don't scratch'. This was, and still is, very difficult, especially when you see a child tearing skin off and bleeding profusely. It also meant accepting without comment blood-stained sheets and pyjamas.''

But another mother comments about her young son: ''If left to himself he has always stopped scratching before too long, as if he had reached a climax. Then it is much easier to help and comfort him than to stop him scratching, however calmly one tries.''

As already mentioned, some parents find it helpful to dress babies and younger children in all-in-one sleep suits at night which cover feet and hands, and certainly cotton mitts can be invaluable on the new born. A child can also be encouraged to rub rather than scratch, and nails should always be as short as possible.

Some parents find the best answer is to distract, and a general philosophy of encouraging all sorts of interests in the child to keep him occupied and busy can make all the difference. One paediatrician's advice to us when our own son was young was to find some special interest at which he was especially good—at which he would be "King"!

This, the specialist felt, would give him more confidence as well as providing a focus outside his skin on which to centre his attention. Our son eventually discovered a great love for singing, and the paediatrician's words have proved absolutely right.

The singing led him to join a choir and take part in school concerts, and this in turn led to plays and drama classes. In spite of asthma he has now taken up the saxophone as well, and his long-term ambition is to be a famous actor! All a far cry from the sad, self-conscious five-year-old who wouldn't go outside to play because people might look at him.

Some interests will have their difficulties. For instance, swimming is healthy exercise and it is fun. But apart from the fact that chlorine may sting a sore skin, even the youngest child may be upset by stares from strangers and questions from other children at a large public pool.

The answer here may be a smaller swimming club where the other members can get to know the child and understand his or her condition. Such pools will often need a lower concentration of chlorine, too, since they are used by fewer people. If a child gets used at an early age to appearing in swimming costume and enjoying water, then there are likely to be fewer worries later.

Similarly, the local cub or brownie pack, football club or athletic training sessions, drama or painting group may be more suitable to start with than larger, more impersonal organisations. If members of a group know your child, they will understand the occasional meeting missed and the parents will be in a better position to explain what the child's rash is due to.

There is no need to over-protect the child with a skin disorder once sensible precautions and care have been taken. The child needs to be encouraged to grow to independence, and equally the parents need to lead their own lives, too. So from the earliest age it is a good idea to get into a routine of having baby-sitters and going out occasionally.

Says one mother; "My husband insists on one evening out each week. Our young sitter copes well and soon got used to the routine. I think outsiders to the family are often better parent-substitutes because they are able to be more objective."

All this will create the sort of happy, secure home atmosphere which will help the child to thrive, with or without improvement in the skin condition. As has already been talked about in Chapter 4, even though a tense and anxious family life isn't going to cause the disorder, it may not help it and may even make matters worse.

When nights have been broken by a baby's crying, when the latest treatment has not worked as well as we had hoped or a condition has suddenly got worse again after clearing for a time, then it can be very hard for parents to keep that calm, reassuring expression in place.

Also as we have discussed, a sense of proportion needs to be kept and parents' demands of themselves have to be realistic. All families have their tensions, their ups and downs and conflicts. A perfectly happy and relaxed home can still have worries about the mortgage or brothers and sisters quarrelling and vying with each other for attention.

But if we can acquire a certain equable, optimistic attitude to a child's skin condition then there is no doubt that this will repay dividends in the long run. It is from parents that the children will learn their first attitudes towards the disorder, and much of what they see reflected in their mother's and father's eyes they will eventually reflect through their own. So however much parents may suffer at times on their child's behalf it is important to try not to show this.

Important, too, is that the child should never be shut away from other people and friends in the outside world, even if on occasion young children do ask unfortunate questions or say something that seems unkind. In fact under-fives usually have no built-in prejudices about appearance, and if both they and the child with the problem skin get used to each other, then much of the unhappiness that can occur in later school years may be minimised.

In *Living with Psoriasis* George Sava cites the case of a little boy with psoriasis so severe that his mother, for what she felt were the best of intentions, kept him cloistered at home and privately tutored to save him the stares and remarks of outsiders. The author however advised that the boy should mix with other children, which not only made him much happier but also improved his skin.

And so to school . . .

Making friends with other children, leading a varied and sociable life, learning new interests, going to playgroup—all these will help the child when he or she eventually takes the biggest step of all and starts at school.

There is no doubt that for the children with a skin disorder or some obvious cosmetic handicap, problems will arise from time to time. But armed with support from home and an under-

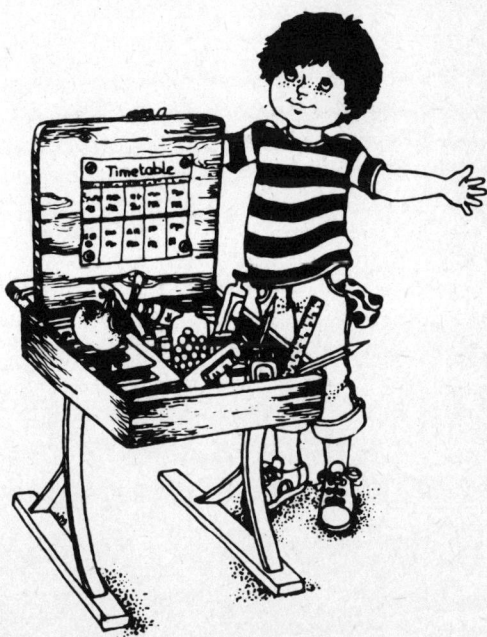

Teachers need to know about special creams and medicines

standing of the condition, the child will be able to deal with these.

Says one adult looking back on her childhood eczema: "I always felt my parents could cope and this inspired me and helped me to cope. They made me feel my value didn't lie in appearances but in my determination to tackle my problem.

"Where I first needed their supportive but firm handling, was in my early school days. They gave me the warm, emotional support I needed and at the same time made me face up to the problem. I was told that other children didn't understand because they couldn't. They didn't reject me, just my skin. At the age of seven I found a true friend who seemed to reaffirm my parents' attitude and my faith in life."

The mother of the little girl with psoriasis already quoted, says: "A child at school has problems that do not bother other sufferers. Most adults can attempt to hide their spots, but schoolchildren have to strip to vest and pants for PE; there is no chance of concealment.

"Moreover this also reveals underwear stained and discoloured by the ointments. I did not want to make Katy different by asking for her to be excused PE so I simply waited to see what happened. Soon she told me she was tired of children asking her why she was at school with spots, and that some of them made nasty remarks.

"As I worked at the school one morning a week I was able to do something about this. Children who came to me for reading would ask me about the rash and I explained that as doctors do not know what causes psoriasis, they cannot cure it. They were very interested in this and thought it rather sad, agreeing to tell their friends that Katy got tired of talking about it. Very soon the subject ceased to be mentioned."

This little girl was lucky, too, because she had both a headmistress and a form teacher who knew about psoriasis and understood how to handle any problems arising from the condition. This is not always the case, and teachers are generally not given enough information about specific disabilities among their pupils, leading to the sort of blunders which can cause more difficulties for the child rather than less.

One example of this was a headmaster who had recently admitted into the school a boy with a large portwine stain on one side of his face. Thinking it would clear up any misunderstanding, the head explained in assembly what the mark was—only to find later that quite a lot of the pupils had not even noticed the birth mark until he drew their notice to it!

Another headmaster, worried that children in a country dance class would not hold hands with a boy with eczema, asked the parents if he could wear cotton gloves. This made the boy feel even more noticeable and ostracised and his general behaviour became increasingly antisocial.

This particular case was helped when the parents went into the school to talk to the headmaster and form teacher, taking leaflets by the National Eczema Society. One leaflet is aimed directly at the children, explaining the condition in simple terms, and the other at the teacher and parent, pointing out the various difficulties that may arise in school.

In it a headmaster says: "A good talk right at the beginning can clear up many misunderstandings that could lead to difficulties later on. Teachers won't think parents are fussing if they go about it in a sensible, unflurried way—and it really does help."

Teachers need to know that a skin condition is not catching. They need to know how to handle itching and scratching bouts, and what to do about any special creams and other medicines the child may use at school. They need to know about special diets or allergies, and how the condition will affect the child emotionally and socially as well as physically. For instance, a child will be self-conscious about appearance when a rash is bad and shows on the face, or embarrassed by the dry skin which in many skin disorders, especially psoriasis, eczema and icthyosis, may flake off on to clothes and floor.

One boy with psoriasis remembers how he disliked the inspection for nits by the school nurse. "Can you guess who had his name taken, while the class watched, not because he had nits but because he had those 'big white bumps of scales which ought to be reported'." More information and better understanding could prevent such a situation arising.

The natural fluctuations of skin disorders will mean that sometimes they affect school activities and sometimes not. When the skin is very sore the child may not want to swim or play games and may feel particularly shy about being seen undressing or in shorts. Concentration in lessons may be poor, and when the skin is really bad it may even be difficult to do something as simple as holding a pencil.

On other days the condition may be almost non-existent and the child able to join in unselfconsciously and happily in all activities. Since these fluctuations are a natural part of the disorders, or of response to treatments such as anti-histamines, parents and teachers have to take them into account when deciding whether or not a child can manage a certain activity.

The NES leaflet finishes by mentioning the delicate balance that exists for teachers between being kind and fussing, between making allowances and giving fair discipline—and this is a delicate balance that will affect everyone concerned, particularly parents.

Inevitably some difficulties can arise because parents are over-indulgent rather than the reverse. Guilt, especially, can make us fall over backwards to compensate for what we see our children as having to put up with, and this can lead those same children to get away with too much!

Yet children with a skin disorder need discipline as much as any others. Without firm handling they can become manipulative, using their problems to shape life how they want it and growing increasingly self-centred. This can also have a detrimental affect on the family as a whole.

"My frustrations about Philip's skin was never vented on him," says a mother. "I couldn't smack a child whose skin was like raw meat, so I smacked his sister instead. 'It's not fair,' she often says nowadays, and she's right—she has at times been treated very unfairly. It is Philip who is the outgoing child who loves life, and Helen who is tense and shy feels cheated."

As described in more detail in other chapters, there are several patient and parent self-help groups which hold discussion meetings on matters such as this, and those who attend much value the support that can come from comparing the feelings and ways of coping. Often a family doctor or specialist will be present to answer questions on the more physical aspects. Health visitors have also been helpful in such discussions, as have other professionals working among those with skin disorders.

Occasionally the tensions within the family or the child may become so intense that some form of psychiatric guidance is needed. One mother describes how this helped her entire family, not just the child with the obvious problem:

"The psychiatrist insisted on seeing and treating the family as a whole and it was at this point that I realised how eczema had affected every one of us, in particular our elder daughter whom I had always thought completely separate from the troubles.

"I had always boasted about how understanding she has been with the bedtime routines. Whereas I spent half an hour or so with the little one, applying the ointments and soothing her, sometimes holding her hands and trying to talk her to sleep, I would then pop into the older one, kiss her goodnight and go downstairs, she never complained.

"Obviously there were many times when the younger one needed a great deal of attention. But the therapy sessions show me that my older child was jealous and even resented me. So I had to try and help the older girl as well as the younger."

Occasionally a child with very serious difficulties, perhaps when psoriasis is accompanied by arthritis, eczema by asthma or when the skin condition is extremely rare and crippling, a child may have to go to a special school or even have a home tutor. Though these courses of action were once normal for any so called "delicate child", they are becoming less and less common nowadays. Even so, there are children for whom special school can be a blessing, since they are no longer the odd ones out and instead are probably the most able-bodied—in comparison for instance with those tied to a wheelchair. Special schools nowadays are friendly, hospitable places, well equipped with interesting activities. If a child does have great difficulties fitting into an ordinary school, one of these may provide the answer, and a list is available from the Department of Education and Science.

Although hospitalisation is also becoming more rare, a short spell as an in-patient can be useful when a skin condition has reached a particularly bad stage. This won't be suitable for every child, since for some the tension of being parted from home and family may even make the condition worse.

But in other cases the rest, the sterile atmosphere and the concentrated treatments available mean that the child improves rapidly. Even though symptoms may return later, he or she will benefit from the improvement which will be good for morale as well as physical comfort.

Hospital can also give parents a short break from full responsibility, which may have become particularly worrying if the condition is in an acute stage. Though plenty of hospital visiting is important and many children's wards now encourage parents to carry out treatments as they would at home, the full burden does not rest quite so heavily and the back-up support from doctors and nursing staff can be very reassuring.

Some parents find that a period in hospital gives them useful insight into treatments and management which they can continue when the child returns home. Says one mother: "During our son's ten days in hospital I watched and learned as if this was my speciality. The specialist took an hour to give us a tutorial on the skin, and this has helped us more than anything before or since."

Another important break for the whole family can be holidays, though like everything else they need to be approached sensibly so that they help rather than aggravate a particular condition. For instance camping and caravanning where there are no baths or hot showers available are on the whole best avoided with the young child, since lubricating and medicated baths are so much a part of most skin treatments. A week or a fortnight without them and a very sore, dry skin might be the result.

If the family stays in a hotel or boarding house, parents may also feel concerned at the idea of bloodstained sheets and pillowcases, sticky deposits left on baths or skin flakes on the carpets. But most of these difficulties are easily resolved. Some parents take the child's own bedding along or use disposable sheets and pillowcases. Baths can be quickly cleaned up after use, and similarly rooms can be swept out daily or vacuumed with one of the small, portable vacuum cleaners which are available.

For the child with obvious food allergies many find that self-catering holidays where you can make your own rules and take your own food to prepare are the best answer. Through the British Goat Society it is even possible to locate local supplies of goats' milk if this is a necessity for the child.

Going abroad is dealt with in more detail in a later chapter, but the problems arising are similar for both adult and child, and again are never insurmountable. One very important point is that the person with eczema should never have a small-pox injection or come in contact with anyone else who has for twenty-one days, since this can lead to a serious virus illness, smallpox vaccinatum.

Other vaccinations when going to tropical countries should be investigated with care—for instance live vaccines are not recommended for those on steroid treatment, and certain vaccines including measles contain egg and animal proteins which would be unsuitable for anyone with an allied allergy. The tuberculosis BCG vaccination is not recommended for someone with eczema.

In the case of psoriasis a specialist points out that though all the usual immunisation procedures may be given, it is worth remembering that a patch of psoriasis may come up at any site where the skin has been injured—for example following vaccination for smallpox or immunisation with BCG.

In spite of maybe having to face a few fresh headaches, holidays are an important necessity not just for the child but for the whole family. In a new setting, perhaps benefitting from sea, sun and rest, it is often a holiday that triggers off improvement in a skin condition, even bringing about the natural remission that most children and parents can hope for eventually.

In the case of Katy, whose story had illustrated much of this chapter, this was exactly what happened. In spite of the rash covering most of the little girl's body, her mother felt they must carry on as though psoriasis was a normal part of life and she took Katy on a swimming course.

"When Katy was six we went on holiday to Norfolk where the sea was very salty. During this fortnight we sometimes forgot to put on the creams but, astonishingly, the spots slowly began fading and receding until only her knees and seat had any patches of psoriasis.

"These areas took months to heal completely but now her skin is clear, although we are both aware that the condition could return. I know we have been lucky, but looking back I feel the experience had little adverse effect on Katy for three reasons.

"Firstly she knew about psoriasis before she developed it. Secondly, the people round her were well informed about it. Thirdly, we did not let it affect our activities. This may be easier for a child than an adult, but when more people know of psoriasis it will be easier for everyone."

The same rules and optimism can be shared by most children with a skin disorder and their families. By taking the right steps we can ensure that when the day comes that a child's condition improves—or even if it does not—he or she will be growing into a happy adult who can often cope better than most with life and the challenges that it brings.

Says one young woman who had severe eczema as a child: "My parents never seemed to treat me as a special case (except where extra physical care was needed). I was gently helped along, encouraged to feel that this was a minor handicap compared with many others. 'O.K' mum would say 'it is a nuisance but one you can cope with. Think of all the things you can do and enjoy'.

"The satisfaction of having coped with a problem is a great strength to me. I feel able to tackle problems and deal confidently with life's stresses. My bond with my parents is an especially close one. They were able to give me the love, honesty and decisiveness I needed, and turned what could have been an unhappy experience into a positive force."

7 — Growing Up

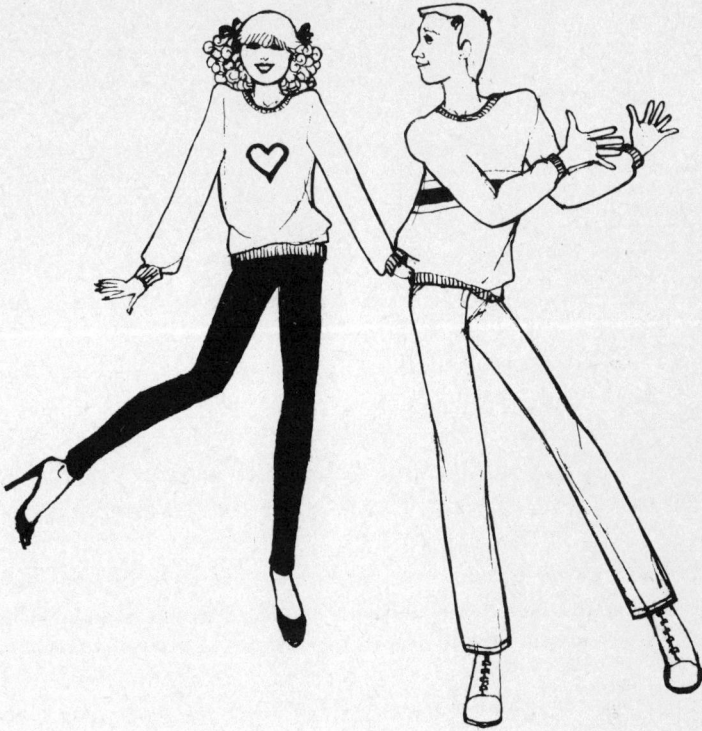

It is important for the teenager to start forming closer
relationships and to feel attractive

"I tried to find a girlfriend partly because of the social
stigma (as I saw it) of being without one and also, and
especially, because I wanted someone to be close to. Having
acne definitely undermines one's confidence in such a
quest. . . ."

Student, aged nineteen.

"I have always felt very badly treated at exam times when
with generally hot weather and natural nerves my eczema
has deteriorated, making exams so much worse and

discomfort, pain and sleep difficulties hampering me from giving a true reflection of my abilities.''   *School sixth-former*

''I think my worst years were in my early teenage, I resented having to wear jackets and short-sleeved dresses when the fashion was for short sleeves or no sleeves at all. But you haven't the confidence to explain what is the matter and tell people psoriasis isn't infectious.''   *Adult patient*

THOUGH no time is a good time to have a skin disorder, the teenage years are a particularly hard period for it to strike. Sensitive about appearance, only just beginning to discover identity and acutely caring of what other people think, the adolescent is especially vulnerable to the social and emotional strains that such a condition can bring.

The cruel irony is that for many this is just the time when skin problems can erupt. The boy or girl who has never had a blemish may suddenly develop the first signs of psoriasis; the eczema that disappeared in childhood may out of the blue make a return appearance; and—most common of all—the feared spots of acne may appear.

In the same way as people think of eczema affecting children and psoriasis adults, acne is mostly pigeon-holed as an adolescent affliction. And even though we have seen from the preceding chapters that it is possible for a baby to have acne and for this condition occasionally to linger on into adult life, it is true that acne predominantly affects teenagers.

One dermatologist who specialises in the treatment of acne concludes that virtually all adolescents have it to one degree or another. In eighty-five percent this is of a fairly minor and easily controlled nature. But in fifteen percent it is serious enough to need treatment from a doctor or specialist, reaching its peak in boys at around nineteen years of age and in girls at eighteen.

Another dermatologist comments that acne is for many people one of the reasons why their adolescence was so memorable and so thankfully past. The appearance of blackheads, and spots just before some important engagement, such as a dance or interview, seems to be an unfortunate characteristic of the disease.

The reasons why acne with its hormonal connections should appear in adolescence, though unfortunate, are on the whole understandable. But why psoriasis, eczema and all the other less common skin conditions that can affect the adolescent should choose to appear or reappear at this particular age too, is not so easily explained.

It may be that hormonal imbalance plays a part in more disorders than we at present realise. It may be that the effects of the changes that take place in the skin at this time are wider reaching than was thought. For instance through the influence of male hormones the horny layer of the epidermis thickens slightly in boys, the pores dilate and there is an increase in the production of oily sebum by the sebaceous glands. The body's immunological system may also undergo certain alterations.

If stress does play a part in skin conditions, then adolescence is a time when anxiety, lack of confidence and moodiness are present in most young people—and if they are predisposed to some particular condition this may act as a trigger. Equally, in an already sensitive person, the condition itself may create such havoc that the resulting unhappiness makes it even worse.

And on top of all this there is the new world of large comprehensive schools, the future to think about, examinations to take, university, further education college or a job to adjust to, plus the growing importance of forming close relationships beyond the familiar world of the family—to say nothing of developing sexuality.

There still are some, as we have seen, who would lay all skin disorders in adolescence at the door of a faulty diet, blaming the convenience foods, the fatty fish and chips, hamburgers and other instant take-away dishes that can fit so easily with a teenager's often energetic and haphazard way of life.

It is possible, as at any age, that foods may be contributing to certain conditions. But since the experience of many has shown that given the most sensible and healthy of diets their eczema, acne or whatever still persists, this would not appear to be the whole answer by any means. Nor, in the view of many who have researched the question, is the teenager's diet so different from that of a child that it would suddenly cause a condition such as acne.

Thankfully most of the theories that sexual repression causes skin conditions in adolescence have gone out of the window—helped, perhaps, by the fact that there isn't nearly as much sexual repression around and yet various skin disorders are as prevalent as ever. This particular theory has always been especially linked with acne, and as Professor F. A. Whitlock points out in his book, the schoolboy folklore that masturbation is followed by acne has added much to the load of guilt and embarrassment that the patient suffers.

> "Puberty is also associated with the developing sexual activity and the complex feelings aroused by its expressions," he writes.
>
> "Adolescence in any case is not the most tranquil period of life and undoubtedly some patients with acne, when subjected to searching psychiatric interviews and psychological tests, emerge as disordered personalities which are then regarded as having a casual relationship to the dermatitosis."
>
> "In the absence of controlled studies of a sample of the population with or without acne who do not attend doctors or skin clinics for treatment, one is in no position to assert that the psychological attributes of outpatients with acne differ in the slightest from those who either put up with the condition or treat it at home as they think best."

Nor, as has already been pointed out in Chapter 4, does Dr Whitlock see that there is any reason to believe that a nervous or anxious disposition causes the acne. Far more justified, he feels, is the belief that the spots in themselves cause anxiety, depression and withdrawal from social life.

Particularly worrying to the impressionable teenage girl may be the hypothesis that over-activity of the sebaceous glands is due to male hormones in the body. She may worry that the reason she has acne is because she has too many of these hormones and may even be taking on male characteristics or changing sex.

But in fact what appears to matter is not so much the *amount* of male hormones in the body, as an individual's sensitivity to them. One dermatologist likens the problem to that of reactions to alcohol: there are some for whom a single glass of wine is enough to make them drunk. In the same way there are people whose sebaceous glands are abnormally sensitive to the effects of male hormones and who get "drunk" on quantities which would leave other people quite sober.

On the whole, treatment for acne, psoriasis and eczema will be the same for the teenager as for the adult, although even more care in the use of steroids and other strong preparations needs to be taken. For instance, in desperation to get rid of sore weeping patches on the face a teenager with eczema might use very strong steroid preparations rather than hydro-cortisone—simply to find that this increases the eczema and further damages the sensitive skin, particularly round the mouth. As a result the whole face may become red and sore.

Though a patchy skin may be hard on the teenager who has never lost childhood eczema or psoriasis, at least he or she will have the advantage of understanding treatment, and will by now have started to find the preparations that suit best. It is at this age that many young people will begin taking treatment into their own hands rather than relying on parents. This may mean experimenting with diet or other alternative treatments such as homoeopathy, or trying some of the hundred and one over-the-counter preparations.

Self-medication is particularly common with acne, partly because teenagers may indeed have been told by family and even doctor that what they have is a passing problem best ignored. At that age they are unlikely to have the self-assurance to insist on seeing a doctor or having a change of treatment.

"You put up with it as a teenager," remembers one adult. "I was fourteen years old when the acne came on. An aunt had it and I didn't think much about it then. No one wanted to know anyway. They just said it was something that would clear up, something I would outgrow. I had spots on my face and neck and gradually they got worse with masses of small ones or horrible big ones. That just went on for years. When I was a teenager I never went to dances. My friends all dressed up but I had all these blessed spots. Eventually I tried everything—different creams and soaps, face packs and herbal cures, eating apples and not eating apples. None of this did any good.''

Though sometimes proprietary brands for acne treatment can work, at any rate for a while, they can simply be a waste of money and at worst they can do harm, particularly if they involve squeezing or rubbing at the spots. Far from healing them, this may instead cause infection and eventually scarring of the skin.

As already explained in Chapter Two, there are now many ways of treating acne including creams and tablets which unblock the pores deep down and control bacteria. As a leading dermatologist in the field of acne points out, this is a perfectly treatable disease and if the doctor is sufficiently enthusiastic and knowledgable about it the long-term clinical effects can be prevented.

But he also stresses that continuous supervision and explanation is necessary, and that doctors must especially emphasise that treatment is safe, and should be maintained for at least six months.

Acne, even more than most conditions, is linked with numerous unfortunate misconceptions over dirt and lack of hygiene, probably because of the general blocking of pores and the black and white heads that result. This leads patients to obsessive washing, sometimes as much as five or six times a day. I recently read a magazine article which suggested the acne sufferers should scrub the face twice a day with a loofah or nail brush, advice which if followed could surely cause an already sore and damaged skin to become even worse.

Though washing and general cleanliness are necessary for the acne patient as for anyone else, this does not need to be taken to excess. The blocked pores that are doing most of the damage are well below the skin's surface anyway and cannot be reached and emptied in this way.

Basic skin care for the adolescent needs to take into consideration the fact that the skin—particularly if there is some disorder—will tend either to be extremely greasy or extremely dry, and probably sensitive to outside influences such as cold or hot weather, wind and even cosmetics and toiletries.

Keeping the skin attractive and in good condition can become a major factor in teenagers' lives, as the questions that pour into the beauty advice columns of the magazines illustrate. "My skin looks constantly grubby. I have developed a complex about it and look down or away when people talk to me," says one girl. "I have a wrinkled look all over my face," I'm begging for help because I am getting so annoyed with people asking if I have German measles," "I am really at a dead end with it," say others.

Two very helpful books in answering questions like this are *Beauty and Medicine* by French dermatologist Robert Aron-Brunetiere, and *Skin and Hair Care* by Linda Allen Schoen. In the first book Dr Brunetiere discusses in great detail the causes of acne and its treatment and also the general care of oily and dry skins. For instance, he says that the vanishing creams thought suitable for a greasy skin actually have the effect of producing more oil since they de-grease the skin and stimulate the glands.

Instead he recommends creams which contain more oil than water—water-in-oil emulsions—and which can be found under the name of "all purpose" or "cold creams" in the shops. When you spread this type of cream over the skin it mixes with the natural fats and so avoids de-greasing the epidermal surface. Consequently, he explains, this cream entails no risk of reactive seborrhoea and to some extent the flow of sebum is stemmed. He also recommends using face powder over this rather than a foundation, and cleansing milk rather than soap and water for the face.

Skin and Hair Care has been compiled from the questions and answers which have appeared in a medical magazine, and covers a wide range of skin care from chipping nails to the treatment of superfluous hair. A typical query comes from a young man who wants to know the best method of shaving when you have acne or any other rash affecting the face. As the book points out, in rare cases the only answer is to grow a beard, but otherwise each individual must experiment.

One dermatologist's tips are to shave with the grain and as little as possible (maybe once or twice a week). If you prefer a wet shave, use a new blade each time; soften the beard by washing carefully with soap and water; leave lather of shaving cream on for at least a minute before starting to shave; after shaving, rinse with hot water, then cold, and apply an astringent antiseptic lotion if this is not irritating to the skin.

The trouble with so many cosmetics and toiletries is that they are irritating to the sensitive skin, and this can create something of a dilemma for the person with a skin problem. Girls in particular will want to make up to hide spots and rashes, and certain camouflage creams can be used by either sex. But by using such cover-ups it is possible to be worsening if not causing the rash.

A lot will depend, of course, on which skin condition you are trying to disguise. In the case of acne, heavy make-up constantly worn may increase the blocking of pores, so when possible (for instance at home when disguise may matter less) the skin should be left uncovered. It is also important that make-up be removed thoroughly at night and never used when the skin is badly infected.

It is also best not to apply make-up to a skin which is sore and weeping from eczema. Since the skin is sensitive, there may be some reaction to irritating substances contained in cosmetics and toiletries. Hypoallergenic products may be helpful when there is a definite allergy, but very often the person with a sensitive skin will simply react to the whole cosmetic rather than to any particular ingredient.

As a dermatologist explains: "Those with atopic eczema are likely to react more severely to irritating substances than do people with ordinary skins. Even compounds which are used by the general population without trouble may be mildly irritating to an atopic. Cosmetics come into this category.

"Unfortunately it is not possible to predict which cosmetic will suit one person and may not suit another. It is only by trial and error that each one is able to find a series of cosmetics which suits them personally. There are on the market whole ranges of cosmetics labelled as non-allergenic, but these are only helpful to those patients who have developed a specific allergy. The identification of such allergies is diagnosed by patch testing by a dermatologist. The so called non-allergenic (or hypoallergenic) cosmetics are then useful to the patient providing that they do not contain the incriminating allergen.''

Since contact eczema is more likely to develop as one grows older, it is worth investigating further if a teenager has never had the condition before and suddenly comes out in an eczematous rash. Worth remembering, too, is the fact that an allergic reaction may show itself in swelling and other allergic symptoms apart from a rash, and that if there is a rash it may not appear only at the point of contact.

Make-up to camouflage patches of psoriasis also presents its problems. ''The main difficulty is that we are individuals with very individual skin colour which is difficult to match,'' says a dermatologist. ''Colour changes with the seasons and what is a good colour on the face may be a poor match on the legs. An ointment which will cover normal skin may slide off or disappear on skin affected by psoriasis.

''Some of the best colour matches can be obtained only by pigments which will irritate some skins, and ointments which camouflage must not run or break up when we are sweating after a dance or running for a bus on a hot day. We must be able to remove them and they must be easy to apply—many patients using camouflage preparations soon get fed up with the amount of time it takes to apply them evenly and to obtain a smooth graduation with the surrounding normal skin. Badly applied camouflage is more conspicuous than the rash.''

Two skin problems which can benefit from the use of make-up camouflage are vitiligo, in which areas of skin are paler than others, and birth marks. The British Red Cross runs a useful advisory service on the use of make-up and correct application and so does an organisation called the Society of Skin Camouflage. Addresses are at the end of the book.

It's Attitude that helps

But supposing, in spite of careful skin care and treatments, a disorder persists throughout those crucial adolescent years and perhaps beyond? It is then that the teenager has somehow to come to terms with the problems involved and, even if only temporarily, learn to live with the condition. Attitude of mind, both of the patient and those around her, once again makes the crucial difference.

It helps if you already have confidence in yourself as a person in your own right, regardless of what your skin looks like or what other people may think of you. But particularly in the early teenage years it is difficult to have achieved quite this self-assured balance. Nowhere is this balance more delicate than in relationships with the opposite sex. For teenagers this is an untried landscape they are venturing into, and it is vitally important for them to feel that they are sexually attractive and acceptable.

Looking back on her teenager years, a psoriasis patient remembers: ''Since starting to go out with boys I have had a lot

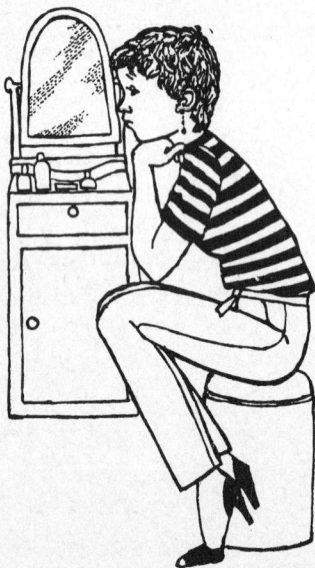

Few teenagers are satisfied with their appearance

of boyfriends, but I always thought that I would never have the luck to get married. Five years ago I met a wonderful man who eventually became my husband and since then I've looked back on my other romances and thought how silly I've been.

"While courting my husband I asked him what he thought about me having psoriasis. We had been going steady for quite a while when I asked him this question, and although I have psoriasis on my hands and occasionally on my face, he told me that it was several months before he realised that I had something the matter.

"At first he thought that I had badly chapped hands. I then told him of my complaint and that I was, at times, covered from head to foot with psoriasis. He told me that I was silly to worry about it and that he wanted to go out with me and not a load of skin.

"Most probably my other boyfriends thought the same, but at the time when I was single and all my close friends were forming close relationships with their respective boyfriends and even getting married, I felt very much alone and that I would never get a chance to marry."

Andrew, aged sixteen, is a teenager who very quickly seems to have come to terms with his chronic acne. It developed when he was twelve and in a fortnight his previously smooth skin was pitted with deep spots on chin and neck. In spite of this he is articulate, friendly and exceptionally confident for his age.

"As far as I know, no one in the family has had acne," he says. "I had asthma as a child, but no skin problems. I do get worried, but I find the worst thing is just to sit around and think about it. If people make comments, then people make comments. Some of the young ones at school will say: 'Here comes spotty.' I just ignore it. It hurts, but there's no point in saying anything.

"I think it helps to have plenty of interests. I go sailing, I'm learning to play the organ and I'm in the school play. I'm also pretty busy taking O-levels at school and I hope to get to university. I play cricket and football and like all kinds of music, including pop."

There are other important factors. He has a close and happy

home-life, and a doctor who is interested in his condition and willing to discuss it with him—though often they sit instead discussing everything else under the sun. After one unsuccessful course of treatment which made Andrew feel generally unwell and did not help the acne, he is now on tablets and a lotion which have improved his skin a great deal.

But Andrew also feels it makes a tremendous difference that he already has a girlfriend, who has been going out with him now for a year. They meet most nights of the week and go to discos and concerts together with a group of other friends. He admits that if he didn't have a relationship with a girl that was going well he might feel that this was due to his skin and become more troubled by his condition.

An educational psychologist who had eczema herself as a teenager now quite often has to help troubled young people with similar problems, and bases her advice on how she felt at that age. Because she knows the unhappiness such conditions can cause she does not minimise their effects but knows how easy it is to lose a sense of proportion.

"I don't think I've ever met an adolescent who was satisfied with his or her appearance," she reflects. "Perfectly normal young people inform me that their noses are too big, their eyes too close together, they are too fat or too thin. Most of their remarks have very little foundation in reality but adolescence is typically a time of self-criticism and uncertainty about personal attractiveness. Inevitably an obvious skin complaint can provide a focus for such uncertainties.

"Another point to remember is that when people feel insecure they often lash out at the most obvious targets. So a girl who is dissatisfied with her own looks may say: 'What's that? I hope it isn't catching.' Bear in mind that this type of reaction is often a sign that someone else is also feeling miserable and uncertain and far uglier than the person they are attacking."

But if, for whatever reason, relationships don't go well, then it can seem like a confirmation of a teenagers' worst fears that people are put off by the appearance of her skin. In the case of Jane, her acne also started when she was twelve, developing into abcesses which left pitted scars on her face and back. She would not take part in any athletic or social event, refused to leave home and finally attempted suicide, so great was her distress.

Between cases like Andrew's and Jane's come thousands of teenagers whose lives may not be blighted by their condition but who nevertheless find that they are greatly affected and who really need support and information.

A few hospitals in this country are now beginning to hold group therapy sessions with young people who are suffering from skin conditions. One hospital in Northampton, for instance, which has pioneered this form of support, found that young people with acne often needed only one or two sessions to feel reassured and better able to cope.

This hospital also runs a series of tape-slide programmes to be seen by individuals and their families. These are informative, with a commentary explaining symptoms and treatments in a factual helpful way. The dermatologist involved says that these days it is quite natural for a fiance, girlfriend or boyfriend to come along to see the programme, and that most go away with a new insight into the friend's or fiance's problems.

Another group is run by the medical social workers at a large hospital in South Wales, and is attended by teenagers aged from sixteen to twenty who have eczema to an extent that needs daily treatment at home and attendance at the outpatients' department.

Reports the social worker involved: "In a safe and relaxed atmosphere the teenagers felt able to let their defences down and to talk honestly about themselves. Strengths and weaknesses were revealed in a supportive and useful way, and a large amount of information was given about the problems associated with the eczema."

He found that discussion of the problems enabled the focus on the skin condition to be a positive one. It emerged that group members had previously felt isolated with their condition, and welcomed the opportunity to talk openly with others in the same position.

Their difficulties seemed to centre around four main areas of their lives—school, finding and keeping a job, social contacts and interests, and the family—and on the whole these problems more typical of most young people with a skin disorder.

At school the kind of conflicts that arose in early days seemed quite often to continue into comprehensive and secondary education. In general the group felt that teachers were ignorant of the problems associated with their condition, and that explanations were rejected.

Some thought that teachers saw them as using their skin problem as an excuse to avoid a particular situation, such as PE. There also appeared to be problems among fellow pupils which members of the group felt stemmed from staff attitudes when situations were not intercepted or controlled. An example of this was name calling that often went unchecked.

The value of group discussion was that on occasion it gave the teenagers a new perspective on their worries. For instance, it did appear to the social workers listening to what they said, that sometimes they read more into happenings than they need, so that a group of children talking and laughing together would immediately be interpreted as discussion about themselves.

"There were parallel situations in work and leisure," they report, "where almost certainly this interpretation was not the correct one. The presence of a skin condition, perhaps not surprisingly made some members of the group very self-conscious and inward looking.

"As a consequence the condition of their skin became an over-important consideration at the expense of other facets of experience and opportunities. Some of the group seemed unable or unwilling to realise that their intense interest in their skin was not shared by the vast majority of people around them."

Similarly, having selected suitable areas of employment, some of the group felt that they were discriminated against in interviews, and that because of that they had to over-prove themselves to prospective employers. Lack of success following an interview made some feel this was due to their skin rather than to some other reason, such as that a better qualified candidate was available for the post.

In social and leisure life, a circular effect could start, so that a lack of friends in the first place inhibited participation in activities, and limited activities and interest, in turn inhibited social contacts.

Socialising generally depended on the condition of the skin, and was determined in two ways—by how the person himself felt at any given time, and by the reaction of others to the way he or she looked. Girls in particular worried about their physical appearance and their attractiveness to boys, feeling that their skin might be putting the boys off from making sexual advances.

Discussion helped the group to see that difficulties in work and friendships might not necessarily be caused by eczema, but by the teenagers' conviction that it was! Some young people, seemed to need to use the skin condition as a focus of their lives, and understandable though this might be, they began to see that over a period of time this could alienate possible friends.

A frequent area of annoyance within the family was the degree to which the routine of family life and functions was ordered round the condition of their skin. Discussion helped the teenagers to see that an exaggerated response to the problem follows only too easily from the practical problems: greasy clothing and bedding, for instance, and extra work and expense for the family. Parents will also be naturally concerned about their child, and this might show itself on occasion as over-protectiveness.

Sorting out the Difficulties

But though discussion with others who understand can give a new and perhaps more constructive slant on the way you look at things, there is no doubt that there are difficulties, and that the sort of problems the teenagers discussed are not only in the mind.

Ray Jobling, remembering his teenage years with psoriasis, says:

"When forced to expose myself I tried as far as possible to stick closely to my friends who were already in the know, and their obvious acceptance seemed to reassure the more curious and suspicious strangers. Possibly I afforded them few opportunities to get close enough to quiz me.

"Away from my protective circle, for example when involved in selective representative sport, I had greater problems of stage management, but early or late arrival for changing, tactical choice of a changing room position which maximised privacy, and wearing whenever possible concealing clothing, all served to restrict the visibility and obviousness of the disorder.

"However, being at school forced me daily into close proximity with others and in situations where it was difficult to avoid exposure at some time or another. Petitioning the staff for special treatment when nerve faltered involved presenting an elaborate account which always ended up with the conclusion that the only possible reason for 'making allowances' was the protection of 'my feelings'. One relied entirely, therefore, on the sensitivity of the teacher concerned . . ."

As with the younger child, it can help for the teenager either alone or with parents to make a special appointment to talk to whoever is responsible for pastoral care at the school, a form tutor for instance or a counsellor. It can also be invaluable to involve the games teacher in any meeting so that specific difficulties in this area can be talked over.

As the educational psychologist points out, skin disorders will flare up at the most inconvenient times, very often just before or during examinations. "With regard to these," she says "it may be helpful to involve the medical officer attached to the school, who can request dispensation from exam boards on medial grounds so that allowances can be made.

"For instance, during a really bad bout extra time may be given, dictating facilities, even a postponed date. So it's important to look into these possibilities."

Careers can also present some very real problems to the patient with a skin disorder, and this is another of the pressures which the adolescent may feel when deciding on future employment. This may not necessarily be because a certain job is unsuitable but because people think it is.

For instance, one eczema patient questions the need to include on certain job application forms whether, along with epilepsy or heart trouble, the applicant suffers from a skin condition. "Had I entered eczema—or acne or psoriasis for that matter—would it have made any difference to my suitability for the post, I wonder?" he asks.

Another psoriasis patient recalls the blow of being turned down for officer entry into the services, even though apart from his skin disorder he was fit and exceptionally active. "It came as a profound shock to be formally pronounced unsuitable solely on the grounds of physical unfitness for an active career involving close engagement with others," he says. "For the first time I saw that it really was going to make a fundamental difference to me . . . I was in effect a different person from the one I thought myself to be."

A specialist who has had particular experience of contact eczema and industrial dermatitis, and is an adviser to the Employment Medical Advisory Service, feels that there are both valid and invalid reasons for the prohibition of certain jobs to those with skin disorders.

For instance, if you have psoriasis or eczema severely affecting the hands, then certain food handling and preparation jobs may be unsuitable. Similarly, if the skin is very sensitive, it may be that without necessarily developing an allergy as such, the person may find that the chemicals used in hairdressing or even the constant immersion of hands in water when shampooing can cause irritation. This may particularly be the case in a new job when the skin has not adjusted to an irritant.

Industrial eczema, caused by an irritant or an allergy to some substance involved in work such as the chemicals in the rubber of car tyres and radiator hoses or the additives in factory oil, can also cause job problems. If any existing allergy is known about, then the teenager must take it into consideration when deciding on a job. But though it is obviously wise to look into all these possibilities, as the specialist also points out, the wish to do a particular job may be so overwhelming that the person will decide to give it a try come what may.

"Such factors make it extremely difficult to lay down any

hard and fast rules about job suitability,'' he says. ''Careers advice should be given often and parents, teachers, school career officers and general practitioners need to be made more aware of the need for such advice—and hospital departments of dermatology and the Employment Medical Advisory Service more capable of providing it.''

Though they may not see themselves as either disabled or handicapped in the usually accepted sense, school leavers with skin problems can also seek guidance and information from the Disablement Resettlement Officer at the Job Centre. If the condition is particularly serious the officer can arrange for the school-leaver to attend at an Employment Rehabilitation Centre for assessment of aptitudes in suitable areas of work.

The school medical service can also play a part, and there are useful forms available which will pinpoint the sort of jobs that are unsuitable, for instance where there are skin irritants in use or where there is a dusty atmosphere. It's a good idea for parents and their children coming up to career decisions to see the school medical officer with this in mind.

In fact, though parents may by now be taking a back seat as far as certain aspects of their child's condition are concerned—such as applying treatment, and dealing with doctor or specialist—their support is still vitally important to the teenager.

The social workers with the group of teenagers in Wales found that in some parents their own lingering guilt feelings about their child's skin condition appeared to create a strong desire to compensate for the prejudices which the son or daughter had to tolerate in others. This sometimes made them over-protective and anxious, and if these reactions became excessive then the whole family was affected.

Parental nagging appeared common in connection both with scratching and the application of creams. Some of the teenagers were particularly upset by frequent references from family and friends to the condition of their skin, feeling that this drew unnecessary attention to it.

Says the educational psychologist already quoted: ''It is often said that adolescents reject their parents' interest and advice. Most teenagers, however, will reveal underneath their superficial rebellion and resentment a desire for understanding and support. Vague remarks such as 'Other people are much worse off' are likely to be treated with contempt. Practical suggestions about make-up, suitable clothes and commonsense suggestions about other aspects of appearance apart from the skin may well prove acceptable.

"But don't expect thanks for such help! The teenager may well initially reject offers of help quite violently, only to take advantage (with elaborate casualness) of them weeks later. It's important for the parent to try not to become convinced that their child is suffering agonies unknown to the rest of the age group solely because of his or her skin complaint. It is often reassuring to talk to other parents of teenagers—all may find they have much in common."

Andrew, the sixteen-year-old with acne quoted earlier in this chapter, is an excellent example of how parents can influence a teenagers' attitude to himself and the disorder. His parents, Andrew says, have always been helpful and supportive.

"It helps a lot if you have parents you get on well with and with whom you can talk things over. I think if my parents had been different I wouldn't have had the attitude I have. They don't go on about it, I wouldn't like it if they did. But I know they are interested and will remark if I'm looking better. I can always turn to them if I'm worried."

As with the young child, the teenager is likely to find that just as suddenly and mysteriously as the skin condition arrived it is likely to disappear. With support from parents, school, friends and the outside world he or she should be left physically—and one hopes emotionally—none the worse for wear.

8 – Coping as an Adult

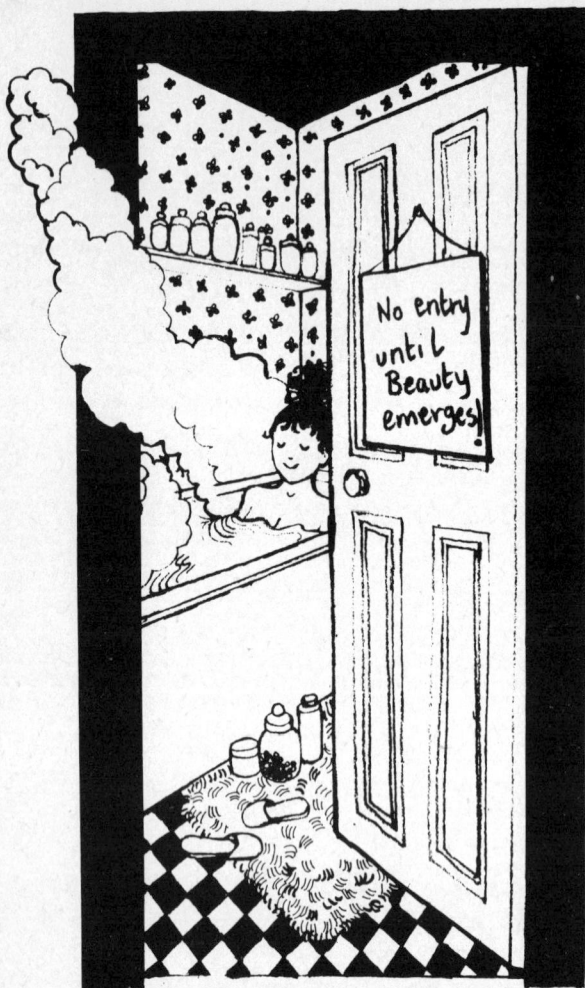

A sense of humour can be a saving grace in any marriage or relationship

"When the spots came back I didn't think it was acne at first because I didn't think you could have it as this age. I felt I had to cover it up or hide myself away. Once you get into that state it overtakes your thoughts."

''How can a marriage prosper if the partner smells, is greasy and crackles every time he (or she) moves? Not to mention occupying the bathroom two hours at a time!''

''I recently obtained a job in the Civil Service and was sent for a medical. Two weeks later I was sent for an identical medical with another doctor. Two weeks later yet another summons came, at which I finally found out that all they were worried about was the fact I had eczema.'' *Adult patients*

HAVING finished the last two chapters on such an optimistic note, it may seem contradictory to launch immediately into the subject of adults coping with skin disorders. But in spite of the fact that many conditions of childhood and teenage years do disappear, some, as we've also seen, may start for the first time in later years or linger on to some degree or another.

The surprise for many people may be that acne can be one of the lingerers. Though in the vast majority of cases it is limited to adolescence, there are some people for whom it is still a problem right into the twenties and thirties, and some for whom it makes its first appearance in middle age, although this is more unusual. Psoriasis can also develop in later life, sometimes as late as seventy or even eighty.

So can eczema. The atopic type found in children and young people seldom remains latent until late adulthood, though it is possible. More usually it will disappear for long periods, some- times never to return and sometimes perhaps triggered off again by a particular factor in a person's life. However, contact and irritant eczema are common in adults, and other types of the disorder can crop up at any time in adult life, particularly seborrhoeic and discoid eczema.

Some other skin conditions will be more likely to occur in a specific age group or phase of life. In pregnancy, for instance, women will often notice a change in skin pigmentation with darker patches developing on various parts of the body. In some women urticaria and pruritis can affect the later months of pregnancy, and in others hirsuteness (thickening and growth of body hair) or alopecia (thinning or loss of hair) may occur.

When such conditions are allied with pregnancy they will usually disappear after the baby is born. It is also encouraging to know that though in certain cases an existing disorder may become worse during pregnancy, in a large number of cases it will improve. One woman whose acne had affected her from the age of fifteen cleared completely during both her pregnancies, and a psoriasis sufferer had the same experience at thirty-three, having had the condition since the age of six.

In some men and women certain skin conditions will be more common in middle age. Rosacea, for instance, can develop for the first time in men and women at this time. As has been said already, but can't really be stressed often enough, the flushed face and sometimes enlarged nose can be very distressing for the patient because people associate it with too much drinking. In fact alcohol along with other factors such as hot drinks and food can make matters worse, but it is not a prime cause. Indeed one dermatologist has had cases which appeared to be related to a dental infection, and which were cured after treatment of an abscess.

Other hazards for the middle-aged woman can be the hot flushes and increases in body hair which may develop in the menopause. Rather like blushing, the hot flushes are caused by the dilation of blood vessels which may in turn be influenced by the general upheaval of female hormones at this time. Courses of oestrogen have been known to help with these symptoms as long as they are thought otherwise suitable for the individual concerned.

Other skin conditions tend to affect the elderly, and these include varicose eczema in association with varicose veins, when the veins become swollen and the blood flow sluggish, and ulcers. Both may have connections with over-weight and hereditary factors, and ulcers can be triggered off by an injury or by an attack of thrombosis when a clot forms in the bloodstream. Pruritis, or general irritation of the skin, may become worse as people get older, and some rashes may be the result of drugs taken for another illness. So these need careful diagnosis.

The reason some of these disorders appear at this particular period of life is the gradual ageing process of the skin. As we grow older the skin loses much of its water content, and the sebacious glands tend to secrete less oil, so the skin becomes increasingly dry. Both the epidermis (top layer) and the dermis of the skin become thinner as less keratin is produced to renew cell growth. There is also a deterioration in the supporting collagen fibres, which results in decreased elasticity and the wrinkling and sagging familiar in older people.

In *More Than Skin Deep* dermatologist Thomas Sternberg points out that though some of these changes are inevitable, the age and speed at which they occur can be influenced by certain factors. For instance, regular creaming and lubricating of the skin from teenage years onwards will naturally keep the skin more healthy and supple and may even help to prevent the type of stretch marks on a woman's tummy that often result from pregnancy.

He also reminds us that a pleasant expression will make a lot of difference to how the face stands up to the passing years! Particularly ageing are the frown lines that form on forehead and between the eyes, and downward corners to the mouth. Keeping alcohol within limits and eating a well-balanced diet with plenty of fruit, vegetables and roughage will also be good for the skin, even if this does not keep any particular skin disorder at bay. Lack of sleep, fatigue and inadequate exercise will all take their toll on the skin as they will on the rest of the body.

But like many others, this dermatologist singles out sunlight as the most devastating factor in speeding up the ageing of the skin because it affects all the layers, including the deep subcutaneous layer, in producing sagging and wrinkling. It produces lentigos, the brown marks which appear with age and are known as 'liver spots', and it also produces the scaly, reddened spots, actinic keratoses which can develop into skin cancer.

He describes girls in their teens for whom the destruction has already started as they sunbathe in their bikinis, and says that the damage is cumulative, permanent and progressive so that the fine tan will come back to haunt them with wrinkles and sags one or two decades later.

But as we all know, right from those early years there are various common-sense measures which can be taken to guard the skin from at least some of the dangers. Before exposure good-quality sun-screening preparations should be applied which protect the skin while at the same time encouraging its natural tan-producing pigment, melanin. Afterwards lubricating and moisturising lotions need to be massaged in.

Particularly at first it helps to limit the time of exposure to around fifteen minutes a day, starting early in the morning or late in the afternoon when the sun's ultra violet rays are less fierce. In particular dermatologists stress that should any actinic keratoses form they must be seen by a doctor. Though not malignant in themselves, if they are left untreated a certain percentage will become skin cancers.

Some skin conditions, of course, are actually caused or made worse by exposure to the sun or simply to the light. Photo-sensitivity can cause various skin conditions which seriously restrict a person's life-style. One woman, for instance, describes how she gets by wearing clothes that cover her whole body, summer and winter, and by using various protective preparations. A yearly holiday abroad is managed only by constantly running from the shade of one building to another.

Warning about the sun, however, may be very confusing to those who know that sunshine is good for their particular disorder—for instance certain cases of psoriasis, eczema, acne and vitiligo. As with any form of treatment or therapy, the advantages need to be weighed against the possible disadvantages, and as long as precautions are taken most patients should be able to enjoy any benefits without coming to harm. They may also feel that the odd premature wrinkle or sag is worth the clearance of a rash or blemish covering the whole body anyway!

The treatments for the adults skin disorders are mostly the same as those outlined in chapter 2, but there are times during adult years when for one reason or another these will need modifying or leaving off altogether. For instance, during pregnancy steroid preparations should be used with even greater care. Though it is quite possible that a condition will improve anyway, if treatment is needed then it is best to stick to hydrocortisone or the very weakest steroids, or to use non-steroid preparations. Systematic steroids (taken orally) should be avoided altogether.

This is because the use of steroids on pregnant animals has been shown to cause abnormalities of the foetus, and though no connection between this and human beings has been established, manufacturers of the preparations recommend caution. It is also possible for strong steroids to weaken and thin the skin, which could result in more severe stretch marks on the stomach and thighs than would otherwise occur.

It is also recommended that whenever possible neither PUVA or methotrexate should be used as a treatment of psoriasis during pregnancy because the long-term side effects are as yet unknown. There is also the possibility that the drug methotrexate could affect the husband's sperm and the wife's eggs, so where this or a similar drug is being given, doctors advise against conception. Ordinary dithranol, tar and ultra-violet light can be used during pregnancy without any worries, however.

As one specialist explains, psoriasis in the elderly is not essentially different from that in younger age groups. Writing in the Psoriasis Association's magazine *Beyond the Ointment* she says:

"However, the affected person may well have acquired other medical problems with the passing of time, and the addition of an extra burden can be trying.

"Moreover, disabilities may actually hamper effective treatment of the skin; certain areas may be out of reach and application of ointment fraught with difficulty for that reason or because of impaired sight. Inadequate washing facilities, a cold bathroom or bedroom or difficulty in getting in or out of the bath will all lead to less than ideal treatment regimes. The dermatologist or general practitioner should try to take such factors into account when prescribing and suggest a treatment programme that is not too complicated or ambitious.

"Sometimes in these circumstances a district nurse can help by, for example, treating scalp patches daily or by applying dressings. Often a relative will come to the rescue and carry out quite complex treatment, for example using dithranol, with care and enthusiasm. Occasionally a spell in hospital may be useful, both to instruct the patient in treatment, and to reduce patches of psoriasis to more manageable proportions."

It's also encouraging to know that it is never too late to try new and successful treatments. For instance, this specialist says that some of the long-term hazards of powerful treatments are less worrying for old people. Methotrexate can be well tolerated if it is given cautiously and the patient is supervised with care.

One old lady with psoriasis writes how hospital did the trick—on her seventy-eighth birthday. "My psoriasis had been getting steadily worse for months in spite of everything I did to prevent it. However, after the kind and gentle treatment I received at the skilful hands of the medical staff, I could see my skin changing back to normal after the second week, and then a short session of ultra-violet light clinched it.

"Even the doctor said it was a remarkable response. But there was something even he didn't know about—something which gave me a wonderful peace of mind I will never forget. On 12th January I celebrated my seventy-eighth birthday in the ward, and 'celebrated' is the right word as the sister and nine of her nurses organised a smashing birthday party with musical honours, a special chocolate birthday cake with seven candles and bottles of sherry, Dubonnet and Martini to wash it down. The girls were terrific. They came into my ward at 7.30 am with birthday wishes, hugs and kisses which left me almost overwhelmed.

"Perhaps the hospital authorities should take note of this 'special therapy' and use it for other patients in future. In my case I think it was the kind staff's social treatment as much as their medical care which brought about my rapid recovery."

Another late starter found that goats' milk was the answer for her—after twenty-eight years of suffering with eczema. "Following advice I read regarding alteration of diet, I switched from cows' milk to goats' milk. It was the changing point of my life. From the first carton, the improvement was dramatic—nobody could believe it, I was a different person.

"It would be wonderful if goats' milk cured everyone suffering from eczema, but it's well worth trying. I only regret that no doctor ever put me on a diet—and yet it's so simple."

For some people it is as they grow older and more used to their skin condition that they learn to keep treatments to a minimum, sometimes abandoning them altogether. "I find the less I think about it, the better I am," says Jane, a psoriasis patient. "I have a theory that worrying about skin, putting ointments on it and thinking too much about it actually makes it worse. It's best almost to ignore it.

"I've also found that since I stopped worrying about the psoriasis it doesn't itch. I've been to numerous skin specialists and tried all sorts of ointments including disgusting tar concoctions. Now I keep treatment to a minimum just preventing any scales from forming. Sometimes I use a steroid cream on patches on my hands, but mostly I stick to a plain cold cream."

Jane is a very good example of someone who has come to terms with her skin condition after many years of living with it. The psoriasis started when she was six and stayed with her right through her schooldays, her teenage years and into adulthood. Yet she has managed to build up an interesting career for herself and has a wide number of interests. Now she is thirty-three, newly married with a baby and in fact the only time the psoriasis has disappeared completely was during her pregnancy.

"I wasn't too disappointed when it returned," she says. "It was gone for such a short time and I knew this was likely to happen. Being clear was just something that went with being pregnant, like growing larger! Psoriasis is so much part of my life now that I rather take it for granted, I suppose. For instance, I realise there are various automatic reactions of which I am not aware any more, such as choosing suitable covering clothes. I make straight for the racks with long sleeved and high necked dresses and I wear my hair over my forehead to disguise any patches on the hairline.

"But that's just so much a part of me, I don't think about it and I don't worry. I have had some bad experiences—I remember once being asked to leave a swimming pool by a uniformed—or uninformed—official. I did, of course, and it put me off going swimming for a while. But now I go again, though I find it easier among a crowd of friends.

"I've been lucky in that I have some very good friends and my psoriasis never seems to have got in the way of relationships. When I was younger I was rather studious anyway and not especially interested in boys, and as I got older I found that by the time a man got to hear I had psoriasis I knew him well anyway, so it hardly seemed to matter. In fact anyone I know I'm not bothered about for a moment. It's the casual people passing or the hairdresser I mind about."

A good relationship

For some with skin disorders it is the more intimate relationships with the opposite sex that cause most problems.

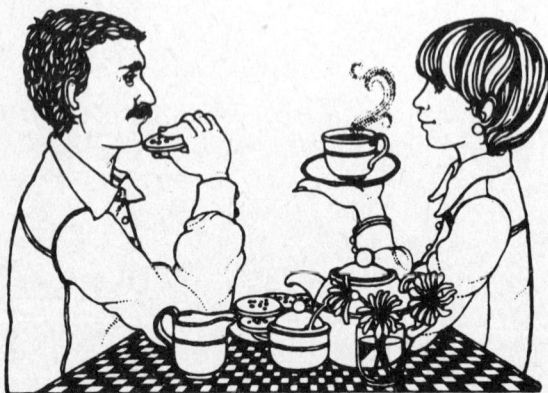

Achieving a harmonious, supportive relationship can help people cope with their problems

As one girl in her twenties, newly qualified with a degree as a fashion designer, found, the return of childhood eczema had a drastic effect on her confidence in herself as sexually attractive.

"Personally I was revolted by my body, of which up until that time I had been extremely proud, having what is regarded as a good figure and naturally tanned skin, which surprisingly is not at all dry. This adversely affected my love-life greatly and even though the eczema has now disappeared I still feel I don't 'love' my body any more—and to this end was uninterested in gaining a sun tan this summer although on a similar holiday two years ago I spent every moment lapping up the sun."

A man with psoriasis describes how in his youth he felt no woman could possibly be interested in him because of the scaly patches that covered a large area of his body. A woman with acne says that in spite of her husband's assurances that a few spots made no difference to him, she felt that he was just pretending and that underneath they must put him off.

Quite apart from appearance, what is often overlooked, is the sheer physical discomfort a skin condition can cause when making love. Many disorders such as eczema, psoriasis and pruritis will affect the genital area and if the skin is generally sore and itchy it may be difficult to get any pleasurable sensations from physical intimacy and even to shy away from touch. Close bodily contact can also make a rash more sore and itchy as the skin becomes hotter.

Add to this the need for creams and ointments and other treatments which may be cosmetically unpleasant, and it is hardly surprising that many skin disorders create great difficulties for a couple when trying to achieve a successful sexual and marital relationship.

The skin for all of us is an important erogenous zone, stimulating sexual response. One specialist lists sexual attraction as one of the three main functions of the skin, yet one that as he points out is not usually mentioned by standard text books. "It must be remembered," he adds "that skin texture has an important role in love play and this is often the real reason underlying the patient's worry about blemishes or rough areas on the skin."

Some of the steps that need to be taken are purely practical. For instance anyone with a rash that affects the genital area should not be shy about mentioning this to the doctor. Sometimes it may be a different skin disorder altogether, needing separate treatment. It is also advisable not to use stronger preparations such as steroids in sensitive areas of the body as these may have the effect of actually making the rash worse.

Looking back on why she thinks her skin condition may have contributed towards her broken marriage, one woman with eczema says: "Living at close quarters with another person, irritability and depression because of the condition of the skin can often be misunderstood by the partner. There is a danger of a vicious circle being set up.

"Add to this the daily irritants over the long period of a marriage, the fluctuations caused by pressures from careers, money worries, hormone imbalances and the bearing and rearing of children and you may find the situation is taxing both partners, though in different ways.

"To other couples I would say—for heaven's sake talk about it and don't lose your sense of humour. It is better to have a grouse or a joke (if you can) than to make the other feel untouchable."

Sense of humour is stressed by various patients and their partners time and again as the saving grace in any marriage or close relationship. One woman with psoriasis was convinced that no one else would want her after her first husband died, yet she eventually met a widower who asked her to marry him.

"I warned him he would be sharing his life with a greasy, smelling individual who went to bed in old pyjamas, and shuffled about the bedroom knee deep in scales. In spite of this he took me on and needless to say I'm very happy. He has a marvellous sense of humour—well, he would have to have, wouldn't he?"

Another eczema sufferer describes her bedtime routine as follows: "To retain some of the mystique I find if the skin is particularly ugly, e.g. when hot in the bath, then a sign on the door—something like 'No entry until beauty emerges'—does the trick. Going to bed with all the goop on—well, a cotton nightie (Laura Ashley's are marvellous), a dash of perfume (on the nightie, never on the skin) quick flurry and the light off and a guy isn't even aware he's next to a blotch.

"So we get by. Sure, sex is not as to the fore in our marriage as we would perhaps like, but we make the best of it. We do love each other and this is just one of the give and take things. Also remember that there are an awful lot of couples we know who to us are beautiful and perfectly normal, who have more problems than we'll ever know!"

For many it is the achieving of this harmonious, supportive relationship that above all helps them to cope with problems connected with their condition and to face other pressures in their lives. Remembers one woman with acne; "I took up sport because I thought it might help and also because I was too worried about my appearance to go to dances and socials. That was how I met my husband. 'What are you worried about?' he said. 'It's just a few spots.' Somehow having him with me made me feel less self-conscious."

The wife of a man with psoriasis described in *Beyond the Ointment* how they have lived with the condition for over thirty-three years since the first patches appeared on her husband's elbows when they were both eighteen years old.

"The patience and forebearance with which my husband tolerates psoriasis continues to amaze me," she says. "I am filled with love and admiration for him as he copes so successfully with the difficulties of everyday life. After several rebuffs at the barber's I became my husband's hairdresser, and remain so today.

"I bless the periods when I vacuum from sheer habit rather than necessity, for this means a quiet period for my husband with little or no scaling. Joy for me is to see my husband looking bright and cheerful and enjoying himself. Like last summer when, for the first time in about twenty-five years he was able to wear bathing trunks and revel in the new found freedom of sea and sun bathing."

The husband of another psoriasis patient feels strongly that facing a skin problem needs to be a joint venture. "I started by trying to tell you how *I* lived with it and ended up by telling how *we* succeeded," he says. An eczema patient stresses: "The moral support of one's partner is vitally important in facing the world in one's social life."

Because of hereditary factors, as has already been discussed in Chapter 6, an important decision many couples with a skin disorder have to face is whether or not to have children. But, apart from types of the condition epidermolysis bullosa where one child born with the condition will almost certainly be followed by another with it, doctors feel that it is not necessary to limit a family. Even when both parents have a disorder, it is still by no means automatic that their children will inherit it.

Other problems that may arise within a relationship or for that matter for a single person are quite practical. For instance, the social worker at one London hospital specialising in skin disorders says that many of her patients have problems with housing, particularly in renting accommodation with facilities for those regular and necessary baths.

One mother asking for help from the National Eczema Society wrote; "We live on the fifteenth floor in a one-bedroomed flat and are so cramped. Also the central heating is on all through the summer and winter and due to having radiator pipes in all the rooms you can understand how very hot it gets.

"However many windows I have open it's still boiling hot and this doesn't help my little boy's skin. You can understand how distressing it is seeing him suffer this way, and the council won't do anything to give us a new place without central heating because we haven't been here long enough."

This family were eventually moved, but help at the start might have saved them that long period of misery. In cases like this it would probably be best to seek support from GP or perhaps a medical social worker attached to a hospital who could then let housing authorities know of a family's needs.

Jobs, too, can continue to be a problem throughout life. In a purely functional way the industrial dermatitis that develops later in life can make a particular job impossible unless some way can be found to get round the allergy in question. The psoriasis, acne or eczema that spreads to an obvious part of the body can make a job that was suitable, such as chef or receptionist, no longer possible. In really serious cases the Employment Rehabilitation Centre may be able to help. The personnel officer attached to a firm, the social worker with a hospital or the family GP may also be able to give valuable support.

A psoriasis patient tells how the condition affected her prospect of job promotion. Having been with her employers for many years she had to go into hospital for a month's treatment. "I told those who needed to know what was wrong with me, and it seemed to be accepted until I was due to get my promotion when I was informed that due to ill health this had been decided against.

"I decided to fight and after a very long time I won. I am now in an executive position, but it has been a hard slog and at one time it was suggested I be made permanently medically unfit and retired on a small pension!"

The widow with psoriasis already quoted had to cope not only with the shock of her first husband's death, but with her condition suddenly becoming much worse. "It was about this time that I was asked by my employers to bring a medical certificate stating that I was not contagious. They were unaware, of course, that I had had psoriasis during the entire twelve years that I had been in their employ. My hands were particularly affected and looked very unsightly, so as requested I produced the certificate, and then hurt and disillusioned I left to find another job."

Perhaps leaving a job may be seen as a drastic answer, but in her case it paid off. She eventually took a crash course in typing and shorthand at a college and at the age of forty-five passed English O level. Now remarried, she works as a full-time secretary.

Getting Away from It All

Holidays at home we've already discussed. Holidays abroad can have their difficulties, but as we've seen can also be seen as therapy from sun, sea and spa waters. Even so, it's best to make sure of certain facts before taking off.

For instance, in case a skin disorder becomes worse when you are away, it is as well to check whether the country you are going to will provide medical attention on the same basis as at home. Leaflets issued by the Department of Health will help and you should be able to get these from travel agents or the local Social Security office. But read the small print carefully, as you may find you are not entitled to any special benefits if being treated abroad for a condition which was there before leaving. Also, since medical treatment abroad can be expensive, think about insurance.

Vaccination and innoculation also needs careful researching and either a travel agent or GP should be able to advise on this. For instance, the eczema patient should not receive a smallpox vaccination and there are exemption certificates available from the doctor to cover this. Other vaccinations may be unwise for people with particular skin conditions, for instance those receiving certain medication or suffering from allergies, so this needs to be talked about, too.

It is sensible to stock up on medicaments before going abroad and to avoid buying skin creams while away. Many preparations only obtainable on prescription in Britain because of their potentially unpleasant side effects, are freely available in some countries. And one other word of warning — when flying take any tubes of ointment or cream with cabin luggage. Aircraft holds are not pressurised and tubes may split open with somewhat messy results!

The other important thing to remember when going abroad is to follow the specialist's advice already given on safe suntanning. The sun may indeed help a skin condition, but not if the skin first becomes burnt and sore. So invest in suitable screening products before embarking on a holiday. As these may take some trial and error to find, start testing in good time.

Make-up and toiletries can continue to be a hazard in adult years, and for a proportion of people allergies can develop for the first time in middle-age. If a reaction recurs several times with symptoms such as a rash, reddening of the skin or swelling, then skin testing by a dermatologist may show up the culprit. On the other hand it may simply be that an ingredient in a cosmetic is irritating an already sensitive skin, and hypo-allergenic products where some of these ingredients have been removed may be the answer. Again, trial and error is often the only way to find out.

As for the teenager, Linda Schoen's book, *Skin and Hair Care* and Dr Robert Aron-Brunetiere's *Beauty and Medicine* are a fund of information on general skin care. The latter has a particularly useful section on the results of ageing in skin and how to help combat this. As already mentioned, the British Red Cross and the Society of Skin Camouflage also run advisory services on make-up and its uses in disguising certain blemishes, for instance the patchy pigmentation of vitiligo and the flush of a birthmark.

For many the best help may come from group discussion and therapy with other patients similar to that already mentioned for teenagers. In Northampton such groups for patients with acne, psoriasis and eczema have been running for many years. They usually start with an outline of physical symptoms and treatments from a doctor or specialist, moving on to discussion of emotional and social off-shoots.

Says the consultant dermatologist involved: "Such discussion cannot of course cure. In itself it does not directly control the symptoms, but in many cases it contributes towards improvement by getting rid of anxieties and helping towards the development of a sensible approach to the condition and its treatment. In effect it helps to reduce the stress element and as a consequence the skin begins to improve."

He found that many of the patients expressed delight and pleasure in meeting other people with the same disability, and in feeling that the intensity of isolation that they had experienced was overcome. Much of the discussion would revolve round the patients' feelings of being judged by other people.

"Although the females felt that the main judgemental threat was from other women, it is interesting to note that the sex distribution in the group was equal, and that the men felt very strongly about the visual disability, even though for them more of the affected skin was covered."

In many countries abroad such group therapy is becoming an integral part of the treatment of serious skin disorders. An important aim of the groups is to achieve what they call ''deidentification with the skin'', which simply means making the disorder less important in the everyday life of the patient. So though groups may start off discussing treatments, clothing and practical problems, as they become more at home with each other patients can give vent to much more personal feelings, such as emotions of shame or anxiety.

Group leaders have found that having voiced these emotions and acquired interactional skills within the group, people often become more able to deal with problems in their daily life outside. They often find they have more courage to go out and mix with people with areas of their skin exposed that before they might have kept carefully covered.

Doreen Trust who is the founder and organiser of the Society of Skin Camouflage and whose own face is marked by a portwine stain, feels strongly that though such camouflage may have its uses, there is also much to be said for not using any disguise. In the society's literature she is quoted as saying:

''Professional and lay people alike have become aware (sometimes alas very dimly) that the answer to disfigurement is not just to hide, but to educate the mind, heart and eye of those who look at these problems as well as those who suffer them. Cosmetics provide a superficial and temporary 'solution' but this disregards the fact that, ultimately, any such solution will only compound the problem and make the situation far worse for society as a whole. The mindless, or well meaning, imposition of a cosmetic mask for life on a child guilty of no sin, is a red herring solution that conveniently absolves responsibilities.''

One dermatologist tells the story of a young girl who once worked as a secretary in the office next to his. One day she asked to consult him as a patient and in the examination room when she removed her make-up he saw that half her face was covered with a port-wine birthmark. A few months later he saw her again in the hall with no make-up and the port-wine stain fully visible. At first everyone avoided looking at her and yet a few weeks later, they all become accustomed to this beautiful girl with the port-wine stain on one side of her face. As he says no-one thought anything about it and nor did she.

One woman with psoriasis found that it was only after she was happily married that she had the confidence to face the world. "All through my school life I had been tormented by schoolchildren who didn't know any better. I had always gone round in summer with as much cover as possible, no matter how hot it was. Now I have the attitude towards the world of: 'To blazes with you. If you don't like the way I am you can lump it.'"

A woman with eczema found that it was her career in publicity that gave her the necessary push. "On one occasion I was responsible for publicising a large conference. My skin looked terrible and I had to face three hundred and fifty delegates. At first I skulked at home and tried to make all the necessary arrangements by telephone, and then I gave myself a pep talk. I wasn't going to mind what people thought or said about me. I put on a long hair piece and dark glasses, and the only thing anybody said to me: 'You look different.'"

In effect these women had "come out". They were facing the world full on, blemishes and all, and telling that world to adjust to them as much as them to it. It's an attitude that requires a great deal of courage and often may come about only after years of living with a particular condition.

It will also only come about with the help and encouragement of those they face.

9 — Help Yourself to Health

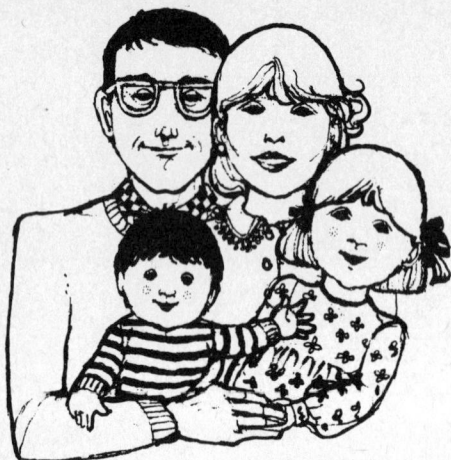

"Here at last were other people whose lives matched ours"

"I didn't know anyone else who had acne. None of my sisters had any trouble. In fact they had beautiful skins, and so did all my friends. I felt the odd one out."   *Susan, aged 20*

"From the beginning I was trying hard to understand my psoriasis and to get information about it. I felt it really would be a help if I could learn as much as possible.

Psoriasis Association member

"Nights are such a misery when you cannot sleep for eczema, asthma and hayfever. Now I think of all the other people who may be awake and desperate and its as though I have friends all over the country."

National Eczema Society member

THERE is nothing particularly new in self-help. From earliest times people have scoured the hedges for herbs to make their own medicines, and remedies have passed from friend to friend and generation to generation. Neighbours used to act as midwives at the birth of a baby, families would nurse each other through serious illnesses.

What *is* new is the recent growth in voluntary self-help organisations in this country. Hardly a month goes by nowadays without a new society starting up to support those with a medical problem, and because of developments in the last few years these now include various skin conditions. There is one umbrella funding organisation raising money for research into the whole range of skin disorders and at least six national groups concerned with specific conditions, with very likely more to come.

Basically all such organisations have the same aims in common. One is to support patients and their families by putting them in touch with each other and providing a point of social contact. Another is to help educate both the patient and the public on the nature and management of the condition. A third is to raise money for research so that new treatments and perhaps a cure for the disorder can be found.

The longest running of such organisations in the field of skin conditions is the Psoriasis Association which started in 1963. Ten people met together with their consultant dermatologist at Northampton General Hospital, Dr Richard Coles, to discuss how best to help one another.

The association now has several thousand members, branches all over the country, its own educational slide shows on various aspects of psoriasis, a quarterly magazine plus other explanatory leaflets, and holds regular conferences and meetings.

The National Eczema Society, in the years since it was formed in 1975, has followed the same pattern. For the first few months a handful of volunteers organised meetings, ran off a newsletter and set the organisation in motion, registering it as a charity. Now, like the Psoriasis Association, NES has a head office and paid staff, even though members are still involved in a great deal of the work and organisation, particularly at local level.

This group also has a quarterly magazine, leaflets on different aspects of eczema including steroid treatment and the child at school, plus one aimed at children themselves explaining the condition in simple terms. There are now society branches in many parts of the country and regular meetings and conferences are held for members.

Other groups are DEBRA—the Dystrophic Epidermolysis Bullosa Research Association; the Maria Scleroderma Therapy Trust; the Lupus Group; and the Tuberous Sclerosis Association of Great Britain. All support patients with comparatively rare skin conditions, but for this very reason are just as much needed.

The need for such organisations is proved by their growing membership and increasing activities. But the help they can give is best shown through the words of members themselves. As is illustrated by the letters that pour into these groups daily, many people feel isolated and cut off with a skin condition, and the first thing they benefit from is the realisation that they are no longer alone.

Says one woman in an article she wrote for *Beyond the Ointment*: "One day I saw an article about Peter who had psoriasis, and the article mentioned the Association. I wrote off for details thinking like so many do, that here at last was the answer, they had come up with some miracle potion to set me to rights. On receiving the reply my first reaction was disappointment?

"But then I thought about it—here was a group of people who like me suffered with psoriasis, but unlike me they were not drenched in self pity. They were going to do something about it, they needed my support, and the support of all sufferers. They did not promise an immediate cure but this Association was desperately needed and I wanted to be part of it. Already I felt better knowing that others faced the same problems as I did, and that someone understood about feeling like a social outcast."

Says another adult with psoriasis: "It was a relief to find that I really wasn't the only one in the world to have psoriasis and feel embarrassed about it. Looking back it's silly to think that I ever thought that my feelings were unique. Listening to other people talk about their problems I was able to say: 'Yes, that's how it is. That's how I feel.' It was wonderful to get it off my chest, and gradually I found it easier to talk about my psoriasis, not only to other sufferers but to other people, too.''

Similarly, one adult with eczema writing in *Exchange* about her local branch of the National Eczema Society says: ''In our experience the benefit seem to be the relief of feeling that one is no longer battling in isolation with one's own eczema problems, and the mutual support which comes from sharing experiences with other members going through a bad patch.

''Several of our members whose children have eczema are in close touch with each other and feel able to ventilate their feelings to those they know will understand and offer practical help with washing, shopping and so on.''

Says another member, the father of a daughter with eczema, who attended the launching meeting of the Society: ''There was a great feeling of understanding. Here at last were other people whose lives matched ours. We were fully aware for the first time that our thoughts and situations were not unique. This awareness by itself was tremendously therapeutic and we found that the sharing of experiences has been of continuing help at local and national meetings we have attended.''

Like this family, many find that the immediate result of meeting others with the same problems and suddenly feeling less isolated is an increase in confidence and an improved ability to cope. Adds the first psoriasis patient quoted above: ''I've formed lasting friendships and my life has changed completely. I gained confidence from the start. For the first time I travelled abroad for my holidays, and have been several times since. I joined a social club and am still a member.''

Says the second patient quoted: ''While previously I just lived in fear of anyone noticing it and dreaded their questions, now I seemed to respond calmly and sensibly. Knowing what I was talking about helped of course, but so did my attitude. My questioners nowadays seem satisfied with my matter-of-fact replies, and really rather interested.''

Says a reader of *Exchange*: ''I read your magazine with interest and am amazed to see that other people suffer like me. I was always alone with my problem.'' And another: ''I was introduced to *Exchange* by my dermatologist, for which I shall always be grateful. *Exchange* has been a great moral support to me, to read of so many people's encouraging experiences and different ideas to alleviate the problems that eczema brings.''

The letters are legion, all showing that it is this moral support going hand-in-hand with increased knowledge and understanding of the condition that makes such a difference. Before, they were mostly in the dark about the possible causes of their disorder and available treatments that might help. Armed with more information they can take an increasing part in helping themselves.

Probably because of the mysteries attached to the whole subject of skin disorders, people who have them can on occasions hold the same misconceptions as people who don't. A survey of a group of psoriasis patients at St John's Hospital in London quotes one man who firmly believed his condition was infectious and felt that if you had a sensitive skin and this was exposed to close contact with someone with psoriasis, you might easily catch it and become infected.

Others felt that the psoriasis spread about the body by a process of auto-infection, others that the scales from one area became implanted in another. One patient whose nails were the first to be affected, and noticed that whenever he scratched his skin psoriasis appeared, attributed this to a germ in his nails and scrubbed them to excess. Even though all these theories are medically disproved, through lack of correct information these patients were needlessly suffering.

Others may lose out on a more practical level. Some patients with eczema struggle on for years without knowing how to mix emulsifying ointment in the bath or that anti-histamine helps control irritation. Steroids are another good example of the dangers of being uninformed. Without correct information on the use and effects of these preparations, patients either may use too much and cause the side effects that people fear, or picking up the odd dark rumour about thinning of skin and stunting of growth may panic and stop using them altogether.

But through the sort of informative articles that can appear in a self-help organisation's publication, or from the talks of doctors and specialists at branch meetings, patients can find out exactly what side-effects of any given treatment may be and how to use preparations correctly so that these can be avoided.

Because of this many doctors and specialists now take an active part in helping the self-help groups, collaborating in the preparation of literature, giving talks at meetings, leading group discussions and deciding which research projects are best supported. Since the layman is not qualified to give direct medical advice, such assistance is essential to any self-help organisation.

In the foreword to the book *Beauty and Medicine*, Dr Terence Ryan comments that even though some established dermatologists have been very suspicious of these patient organisations, most have begun to realise that in a country where the professional has insufficient time to meet even serious demands, laymen can themselves organise a great deal.

Unfortunately some doctors continue to think of such organisations as doctor-bashing pressure groups and to feel that it is not for the patient to be informed on medical matters. There is evidence, anyway, that some feel skin conditions are a trivial form of ailment that the patient should simply put up with. "They'll be starting a society for the common cold next", said one GP when he heard a group was formed to help eczema patients.

"My doctor treats it all as a bit of a joke," writes one distressed mother of an equally distressed three-year-old boy who is covered from head to foot in eczema. "When I questioned the safety of steroid ointments my doctor literally bit my head off, saying he wished people wouldn't read about such medical things," says another mother.

In *Medical Encounters* Ray Jobling writes at some length of the various difficulties that he has had since developing psoriasis as a teenager in what he calls his "career of patienthood". Not least among these was the succession of doctors and hospital staff that changes either in his life or theirs necessitated, but which meant having to rely on his medical notes and a few standard questions for assessment and treatment of his case.

This also often meant that there was no single, constant

individual with whom he could build up a sufficiently close relationship to broach difficult questions. He goes on to describe how in spite of growing pessimism about his condition and available treatments, his career as a patient was grounded in the belief that in due course relief and remission would come.

"The basis of this fiction was undermined by the declaration of a doctor, essentially in contradiction of earlier advice, that: 'Like everyone else with psoriasis you have got to accept that you will have to put up with it for the rest of your life.' This announcement confirmed the prospect of a long-term chronicity and demanded some psychological and social reorganisation. Nonetheless, lacking counselling and sophistication, I still failed to recognize the full implication."

However, on starting at university which meant another move and a new GP and dermatological clinic, the picture brightened.

"My new GP showed a greater knowledge, interest and readiness to respond to questions. He recognised the complexity of the coping problems and was articulate about the relationship between the sufferer's attitudes, his social situation and the course of the illness . . .
"Clearly his level of knowledge and conception of his practice differed greatly from the doctors I had seen previously. It is essential, too, not to ignore the fact that I had by now acquired more experience of the illness and dermatological patienthood and therefore my relationship to the doctor might be said to have changed."

In fact the informed patient or parent can have a far more constructive and positive relationship with the family doctor or skin specialist than the one who blindly follows orders. As one GP admits himself, unless they take a particular interest in the subject, most doctors receive very little training in dermatology as a matter of course. If the patient understands his or her condition and which treatments are beneficial it can be a great help to the doctor.

Within a self-help group the benefits can be two-way. Though there is a place for healthy criticism of those in the medical profession who perhaps are not doing all they could, through the society publications the doctor's point of view can be put as well. Doctors, after all, can also feel frustrated when treatments don't work, causes can't be found or there is too little time to talk properly.

One family doctor, for instance, explains in *Exchange* that though he is a great believer in keeping his patients in the picture about their health, illnesses and treatment this is not as easy as it sounds, particularly in the one-to-one contact which occurs in a normal medical consultation, in surgery or a hospital out-patients' department. Instead he finds the patient groups for acne, psoriasis and eczema patients and parents that he runs far more useful.

"First there is the time factor," he explains. "In a group we are able to spend much more time giving information about the condition and what we are aiming at in our management of the problem, and of course there is always much more time to answer questions.

"Secondly, in a group the patient's role and his image of the doctor's role alter. In the one-to-one consultation of clinic or surgery, the doctor is often looked upon as the authority figure and the patient subservient, whereas in the group the relationship is much more that of equals.

"This leads to a much franker discussion of the problem and more freedom to mention those things which one 'would never bother the doctor with' but which are nonetheless very important to the patient and his family. In the group it is also much easier for the patient to teach the doctor as well as the doctor teach the patient. So both sides benefit."

In the same way articles describe the role of other professionals working with skin conditions, such as the psychologist and psychiatrist, the medical social worker, the health visitor, the teacher, and even the pharmacist, and how the patient and his family can find help from them.

Says the pharmacist:

"A good time to talk over problems is often the late morning or the early afternoon, but whatever the time of day the pharmacist will see you if you ask and give you the benefit of his advice. Your pharmacist can give you straightforward information on how to take or apply your medicine, the times of day at which you do it, the best method of storage, and if any precautions such as avoidance of alcohol are necessary."

The role of the medical social worker may be even more unknown to the patient, since many hospitals still don't employ them within the skin department. Derek Gay, whose group with teenagers at a Cardiff hospital has already been described, writes about the way in which social workers can be generally helpful as follows:

"Although patients are offered an opportunity to talk with me for a variety of reasons, their problems fall into two main groups." he explains. "The first is practical. For example, for children there are difficulties with school or with friends, for adults unemployment, or as a result of their skin condition, problems arising in employment.

"Sometimes one encounters a need for rehousing where a current house does not have a shower or bathroom. Advice may also be necessary over prescription charges and the obtaining of a 'season ticket' for multiple prescriptions. The second group of problems is often less obvious and partly for this reason more difficult to solve. I would group these under the general heading of 'emotional and intangible' problems."

In this category would come many of the emotional problems stemming from a skin condition we have discussed in this book so far, and in this case the social worker would act as a counsellor, listening to the worries and helping the person come up with some solution.

Such help can by force of circumstances be limited, however. To see a medical social worker you have to be a patient at the hospital he or she is attached to, and since as yet social workers are by no means common to skin wards, even when in hospital the patient is unlikely to receive this support.

Exchange of Information

This is where the self-help groups are fulfilling a new and invaluable service. The Psoriasis Association, for instance, was the innovator of the type of group therapy with family doctor or specialist which has been described several times in this book and which gives such invaluable support in discussing problems and finding solutions. Now the National Eczema Society is planning its own counselling service, with social workers giving the sort of non-medical advice which is often as badly needed as the prescriptions for creams and ointments.

Also there are often discussions at local group meetings where patients can pass on the sort of tips about management and treatment which otherwise could come only from long-term trial and error. Parents and patients not only talk about broken nights of sleep or worries over appearance, but where to get cotton socks or a milk substitute.

One psoriasis patient will tell another about the benefits of his or her holiday in the South of France, or about a particular

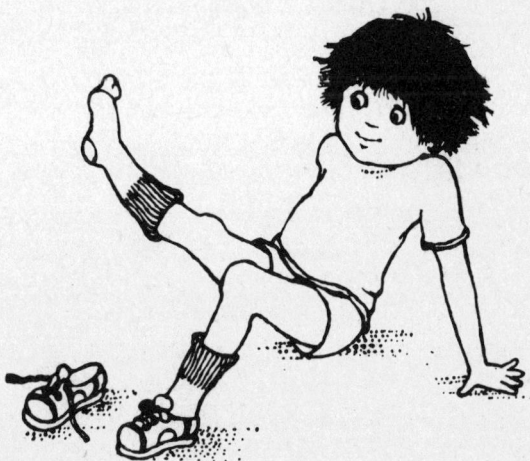

Parents and patients can exchange all sorts of tips, from what washing powder to use to where to find cotton socks

preparation that has worked wonders for his scalp. Through her local meetings one mother of a child with eczema found out about homoeopathy, another about a vegetarian diet.

This exchange of useful information can go on through the pages of the self-help organisation's publications, too. Patients will send in holiday addresses, advice on washing powders and rinsing clothes, pleasant recipes for those on a special diet. One woman describes how in spite of various allergies and skin problems she has successfully had her ears pierced, another how olive oil has helped her cracking nails.

Another aspect of self-help is that together as a group the patients can form a solid body to influence outside opinion, particularly through the various media. Unfortunately this can work both ways, and detrimental publicity can set the clock back further, spreading wrong information and harmful myths. For example not so long ago one article in a national newspaper described how a rugby player had "caught" eczema from another member of his team.

Other old wives' tales too often perpetuated by uniformed reporters in the media are that skin disorders are all due to nerves, bad diet or sexual deprivation. "If people stopped feeding babies junk food there would be an end to skin troubles", said one article in a national woman's magazine. "Invariably those women who have an unsatisfactory love life or are unable to experience orgasm are most likely to suffer from nervous skin complaints like eczema, adult acne and psoriasis," said another recently.

One person writing in to refute such nonsense might not be taken seriously, or might even be regarded with some suspicion as someone with an axe to grind. But a self-help group with the grander title of society or association will make more impact and rightly so, since most acquire a huge wealth of information and experience in their particular fields.

Similarly articles in hairdressing or swimming bath journals explaining the problems of skin disorders increase understanding among people working in these places. In time this should lead to less worried faces in hairdressing saloons and fewer people being asked to leave swimming pools for fear their rash is catching.

Another important area where publicity can help is in education, and one article explaining the difficulties of eczema which appeared in *Where*, a leading educational magazine, is now the leaflet which NES give to schools and parents. Such help is again two-way. Not only will patients and parents benefit, but so also will the teacher who often has to contain children with a varied number of medical problems in the class without extra help or special training.

Of course it isn't just people working among those with skin conditions who need to be reached, but the man and woman in the street many of whom as we have seen may still regard these disorders with the same sort of fear that was once reserved for lepers. Since the start of the various self-help groups the number of articles appearing in national and regional papers has mushroomed, and there have been radio phone-ins and television programmes.

One women's-page journalist described her visit to a skin department of the local hospital. She writes about the woman suffering from Raynaud's disease, which means that if she is exposed to a temperature of less than sixty degrees she goes numb; the little boy who can't sleep because of his eczema; the old lady in constant pain with a leg ulcer. "Words for once finally fail me," she concludes. "Its been an eye-opening experience."

Another way that self-help organisations can influence public opinion on a wider scale is to act as a pressure group to alter legislation or influence change. For example, the Psoriasis Association have campaigned for free prescriptions for chronically ill skin patients, and the NES petitioned for better instructions for use on the packaging of steroid preparations.

They have protested at the possible closure of one skin hospital and at the planned move for another, which could have drastically affected service to patients and research work being done there. Both groups have also been pushing for more detailed training in dermatology for GPs and more research into skin disorders.

As Professor Malcolm Greaves of the Institute of Dermatology has pointed out in the pages of *The Lancet*, research in the field of dermatology still lags behind that in other areas of medicine and dermatological research abroad.

> ''Research into the structure and function of the normal skin and into skin diseases has clearly been inadequate in comparison with the outstanding advances in other branches of medicine. Nevertheless important progress has been made, sometimes as a by-product of research in a different field. There are therefore good grounds for believing that increased dermatological research would not only benefit those with skin disease, but might also lead to advances in other areas of medicine.''

Professor Greaves cites as the main reason for this lack of research the parallel lack of academic skin departments. There are only two in England and Wales, in contrast with Europe and America where a much higher proportion of teaching centres offer adequate facilities. This has the consequences that young dermatologists in training see little career opportunity in skin disease in the United Kingdom, and many go abroad.

However, in recent times the Medical Research Council has renewed dermatological research and repeated its intention to encourage its development. In addition two research departments, one at the Institute of Dermatology, have been organising training schedules for research workers in dermatology and eventually hope to provide more research units.

Reasearch Gives Hope

Meanwhile there has over recent years been encouraging work done in many fields, investigating both causes and treatments. For instance, one project team has been looking into the measurement of itch and the drugs which influence it. They devised scratch meters rather like watches, which could be worn on wrists and ankles and would record all movements, providing a record of the activity of the limb concerned.

In psoriasis, a great deal of work is going on into various

aspects of the disorder. For instance, the most obvious feature in the scaly patches on the skin of someone with psoriasis is the greatly increased rate of cell turn-over in the outer layer, the epidermis, and this increase has been found to be present—though to a lesser degree—in the uninvolved skin as well.

How far this is due to an accleration in the speed to which individual cells are reproduced is uncertain, but it is now becoming clear that there is an abnormally high proportion of reproducing cells in the epidermis of people with psoriasis compared with that of those who do not have the condition. Much present research is therefore trying to establish what controls the activity of these cells in the skin of non-sufferers so that work can be done to identify what is different in psoriasis.

Another important area of research in almost all skin conditions is investigation into the hereditary aspects. In psoriasis, for instance, it has become evident that people with combinations of certain distinctive features in some of their white blood cells (genetic markers as they are known) are over one hundred times more likely to develop the condition than others.

Research continues all the time into new methods of treatment. For example, although PUVA and psoralens are being used to a limited extent already in the treatment of psoriasis, there is a great deal of research needed before the long-term effects can be established. Similarly the long-term effects of steroid preparations on the body as a whole and the skin in particular are still being looked into, and alternative preparations always being investigated.

An example of this is the use of sodium cromoglycate, already so successful in the treatment of asthma and hayfever as the active ingredient in sprays such as Intal. Now research is going on into using this drug in ointment form for eczema, its advantage that it may prevent the itch as well as helping to repair the damage done by inflammation and scratching. Various studies into the uses of sodium cromoglycate have been carried out with children and are still continuing.

Recently interest has also revived in the use of primrose oil for controlling atopic eczema. In 1933 it was reported that children with eczema had a low blood level of unsaturated fatty acids and various dietary supplements were tried including the oil extracted from the evening primrose which is a rich source of linolenic acid. With the advent of steroids such treatment became outmoded, but some more recent studies have shown that patients can benefit from the use of the oil.

Also very helpful is research going on into the use of retinoids. Retinoids are chemical variants of Vitamin A, which is one of the skin's natural controlling factors in the growth of cells and their capacity to produce materials such as keratin, the horny material of the skin. Of the thousands of chemical substances which can be derived from Vitamin A now being investigated, retinoids are proving to be useful in treating both psoriasis and acne.

Exactly how retinoids work in psoriasis is still being debated, although some research workers are putting great emphasis on their immunological effects, i.e. the way in which they act upon the body's system of resistance to attack by threatening organisms. In acne it seems that retinoids work by drying up the excretion of oil glands in the skin, and in one American study almost totally cleared the spots of forty-seven severely afflicted patients. Now similar studies are being carried out in this country and the feeling of consultants involved is very optimistic.

They point out, though, that at this stage these treatments are availabe only on a research basis and not yet approved for ordinary widespread use. They also stress that retinoids are not identical to Vitamin A, which can be a dangerous toxic substance if taken in excess. Our bodies receive an adequate supply of this vitamin in our daily food intake and no supplement should be necessary.

Some radical new treatments are past the research stage and in certain hospitals are in regular use. Laser therapy, which is a form of intense light beamed on to the skin, is now available in this country and is proving successful in removing some of the types of portwine birthmark. Test trials can be done when a child is as young as six or seven and the darker the stain the more successful the treatment will often be. But this is still an investigative form of treatment and available only on a limited basis.

Also still at the investigative stage but becoming widely practised among eczema patients is the method of dietary treatment being pioneered by the Institute of Child Health. As already mentioned in other chapters, it has been found that "at risk" babies whose parents suffer from atopic ezema are less likely to develop the condition if they are breast fed, kept off cows' milk and away from any of the more common allergy provoking substances.

The Institute of Child Health project was the first to be supported by the National Eczema Society when they started a fund specifically for research. More recently the society has given further donations to other research projects, including one on the long-term study of the natural history of infantile eczema and another on cell formation in the skin.

Since it started the Psoriasis Association has given many thousands of pounds to research projects of all sorts. Most recently it has contributed a great deal towards investigations into the use of PUVA, and also steroid preparations. There is also long-term support for a project which is examining the connections between prostaglandins—a group of body chemicals produced in the lower layers of the skin during inflammation—and psoriasis.

The Skin Disease Research Fund has made its first allocations to research in dermatology. A total of over ninety thousand pounds will be supporting a variety of projects including studies of dermatitis in the rubber industry, diffuse hair loss in young women, the various skin disorders of pregnancy and bacterial infection in patients with atopic eczema.

Of particular interest is the fact that a large donation is going towards a project which will be studing the whole concept of skin disorder as a handicap. In all, three thousand patients will be questioned and their disability compared with that of other illnesses and conditions.

Says the dermatologist involved: "Dermatology cannot

compete with acute medicine and surgery which is so often life threatening, but it deserves a fair share of resources provided for chronic disabling diseases. This is because skin diseases reduce a person's capacity to achieve personal and economic independence quite as much as many other disabilities.

"If when pleading for resources dermatology were to use the same language as others it would soon be seen that skin diseases are a very significant handicap to the individual and that they account for a greater number of persons failing to achieve their maximum potential, personal and economic capacity than any other group."

Another important step has been the setting up by the Disabled Living Foundation of a working party to look into the daily living problems of those people affected by chronic skin conditions. The plan is that the Foundation will act as an information service, filling those gaps that still exist in giving support to those who need it and advice where necessary. The various self-help organisations have all been helping in this project, plus dermatologists and others professionally involved in the care of patients with skin disorders.

For many it is progress like that instanced in these last two projects, and the knowledge that research is continuing and that individuals can help by raising money towards it, that is the most worthwhile aspect of self-help in health. From the children who raise a few pounds at their own garden party, to the branch or individual who makes hundreds at a social evening or raffle, it is a positive contribution that brings encouragement in the present and hope for the future.

Says one adult with eczema who came to the society desperate and finished setting up a local branch in her home town: "Members who are participating feel it gives an important sense of purpose to be actually doing something to help shed new light. In my case, belonging and coming into contact with other patients brought home to me very forcibly how mild is my own eczema. For me it has put things into perspective."

Says a psoriasis patient who helped set up a branch of the Psoriasis Association in another town and would like to see every sufferer a member: "They will, I hope, come to see that it's not so much what's in it for themselves, but instead will think of tomorrow's children. An impossible dream, you may think. Not really—I believe that in all men unselfishness lies dormant. Pause and think what we already owe to, say, Louis Pasteur for instance, or Madame Curie and countless others throughout medical history.

"It may be that we will never see a breakthrough in our lifetime, but we are in at the beginning, our puny efforts helped tomorrow's children to wear sleeveless clothes, have their hair done at Raymond's and to be film stars."

One day we would all like to see the mysteries and misunderstandings connected with skin disorders clear, and to hear that cause and cures have been found. Meanwhile by joining together to reach that goal, people are helping themselves and others to learn to live with their condition now, fully and peacefully and with hope.

Acknowledgements

In the preparation of this book, the author wishes to acknowledge the inclusion, by kind permission, of quoted extracts from the following publications:

Medical Encounters by Gordon Horobin and Alan Davis published by Croom Helm Ltd., London (Chapters 1,2,7,9)

Psychophysiological Aspects of Skin Disease (1977) by Professor F. A. Whitlock MD, FRCP published by Lloyd Luke (Medical Books) London (Chapters 4,5,7)

Skin Care (1975) by Dr Bethel Solomon MA, MD, FRCPI, published by Priory Press Ltd. (Chapters 2,4)

Essentials of Dermatology (1979) by Dr J. L. Burton MD, BSc, FRCP published by Churchill Livingstone, Edinburgh (Chapter 4)

Dermatology — an Illustrated Guide (1973) by Dr Lionel Fry BSc, MD, MRCP, published by Update Publications Ltd., London (Chapter 5)

A Guide to Alternative Medicine by Donald Law published by Turnstone Books, London (Chapter 5)

British Journal of Dermatology (1975) 93,111 "The Psoriasis Sufferer in the Community" by Dr R. B. Coles MB FRCP and Dr Terence J. Ryan DM, MA, BM, B.Ch, Oxon, FRCP (Chapter 1)

The Lancet, April 9th 1977 "Dermatological Research in Great Britain: A Reappraisal" by Professor Malcolm Greaves MD, PhD, FRCP (Chapter 9)

Beyond the Ointment published by The Psoriasis Association (throughout) and *Exchange* published by the National Eczema Society (throughout)

OTHER USEFUL BOOKS TO READ:

Living With Your Psoriasis by George Sava published by New Horizon

More Than Skin Deep (1970) by Dr Thomas Sternberg, published by Doubleday and Company Inc. New York

Stigma: Notes on the Management of Spoiled Identity (1968) by Erving Goffman published by Penguin Books

Dry Skin and Common Sense (1978) by Dale Alexander published by The Windmill Press, Surrey

Beauty and Medicine (1978) by Dr Robert Aron-Brunetiere published by Jonathan Cape, London

Skin and Hair Care (1978) by Linda Allen Schoen published by Penguin Books

Not All In the Mind (1976) by Dr Richard Mackarness published by Pan Books

HELPFUL ORGANISATIONS TO CONTACT:

Many of these publish useful further information, leaflets and periodicals. To obtain details send stamped addressed envelope to the following addresses:

The Psoriasis Association, 7 Milton Street, Northampton NN2 7JG

The National Eczema Society, Tavistock House North, Tavistock Square, London WC1H 9SR

Disabled Living Foundation (covering all conditions) 346 Kensington High Street, London W14 8NS

The Skin Disease Research Fund c/o St John's Hospital for Diseases of the Skin, 5 Lisle Street, Leicester Square, London WC2H 7BJ

The Lupus Group, Arthritis Care, 6 Grosvenor Crescent, London SW1X 7ER

Dystrophic Epidermolysis Bullosa Research Association, 38 Cornwall Avenue, Clayton, Newcastle-under-Lyme, Staffordshire

Maria Scleroderma Therapy Trust, 11 Warrender Road, Chesham Bucks HP5 3NE

Tuberous Sclerosis Association of Great Britain, Church Farm House, Church Road, North Leigh, Oxford OX8 6TX

British Homoeopathic Association, 27a Devonshire Street, London W1N 1RJ

British Goat Society, Rougham, Bury St Edmunds, Suffolk

Vegan Society Ltd., 47 Highlands Road, Leatherhead, Surrey

Vegetarian Society, 53 Marloes Road, Leatherhead, Surrey

Coeliac Society, PO Box 181, London NW2 2QY

National Institute of Medical Herbalists, 148 Forest Road, Tunbridge Wells, Kent TN2 5EY.

The British Acupuncture Association, 34 Alderney Street, Westminster, London SW1V 4EU

MASH (Milk Allergy Self Help), 113 Elsinge Road, Enfield, Middlesex EN1 3PE.

Hyperactive Children's Support Group, 59 Meadowside, Angmering, Littlehampton, West Sussex

Foresight (The Association for Promotion of Pre-Conceptual Care) Woodhurst, Hydestile, Godalming, Surrey GU8 4AY

Action Against Allergy, 43 The Downs, London SW20 8HG

British Red Cross Society Beauty Care and Cosmetic Camouflage, (contact local branches of British Red Cross)

Society of Skin Camouflage, Wester Pitmenzies, Auchtermuchty, Fife, Scotland

Index